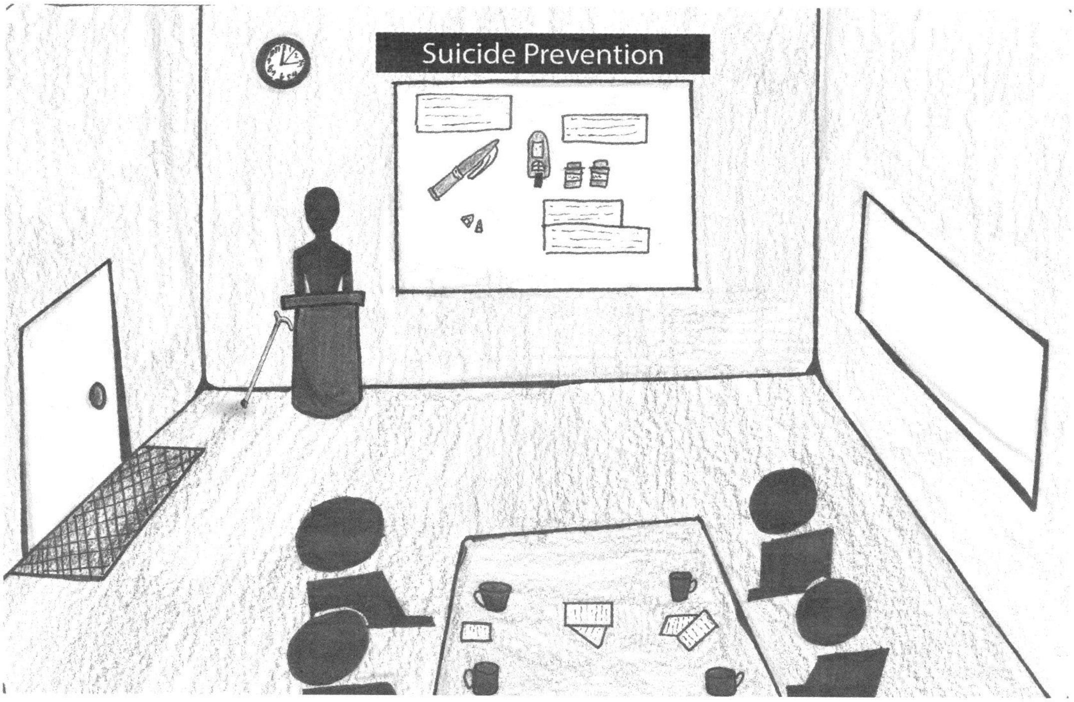

ᒑᒃ ᐅᑎᕁ ᐅᑎᐹᒋᒧᐎᓐ ᐙᔛᓂᐲᐦᒡ ᐅᐦᒌᐤ
ᒑᒃ ᐊᑕᕁ ᐅᑎᐹᒋᒧᐎᓐ, ᐙᔅᐙᓂᐲᐅᐄᓅ
L’histoire de Jack Otter de Waswanipi
The Story of Jack Otter of Waswanipi

Told by Jack Otter
Written by Ruth DyckFehderau
Translated into Northern East Cree by Luci Bobbish-Salt
Translated into Southern East Cree by Louise Blacksmith
Translated into French by Valérie Duro

ᒥᔨᐱᒫᑎᓰᐅᓐ ᐊᓅᓅᑭᒋᐦᑖᑭᓅᒡ
CONSEIL CRI DE LA SANTÉ ET DES SERVICES SOCIAUX DE LA BAIE JAMES
CREE BOARD OF HEALTH AND SOCIAL SERVICES OF JAMES BAY

Funding for this publication was provided in part by Health Canada. The opinions expressed in this publication are those of the storyteller and do not necessarily reflect the official views of Health Canada or of the Cree Board of Health and Social Services of James Bay.

First printing, 2020. Printed and bound in Canada by Houghton Boston Printers, Saskatoon, Saskatchewan. Distributed by Wilfrid Laurier University Press / wlupress.wlu.ca

Set in Verdana font, chosen for its readability. Printed on paper that is Forest Stewardship Council-certified with post-consumer recycled fibres, and that is acid- and chlorine-free.

Cover design by Nicole Ritzer, based on an original design by Cameron Mosimann. Photograph of Mistissini burnt forest (reversed) taken by David DyckFehderau.

Title page illustration by Jared Linton of Mikw Chiyâm Arts Concentration Program, Voyageur Memorial High School, Mistissini, QC.

Published by Cree Board of Health and Social Services of James Bay
Contact: Paul Linton, 168 Main St, Mistissini, QC, Canada, G0W 1C0 / (418) 923-3355
creehealth.org / sweetbloods.org

Library and Archives Canada Cataloguing in Publication

Title: Chaak utir utipaachimuwin waaswaanipiihch uhchiiu = Chaak atar utipaachimuwin, waaswaanipiiuiinuu = L'histoire de Jack Otter de Waswanipi = The story of Jack Otter of Waswanipi / story by Jack Otter ; translator Northern East Cree, Luci Bobbish-Salt ; translator Southern East Cree, Louise Blacksmith ; translator French, Valérie Duro ; writer, Ruth DyckFehderau.

Other titles: Chaak atar utipaachimuwin, waaswaanipiiuiinuu | Histoire de Jack Otter de Waswanipi | Story of Jack Otter of Waswanipi

Names: DyckFehderau, Ruth, author. | DyckFehderau, Ruth Anne, 1967- Story of Jack Otter of Waswanipi. | DyckFehderau, Ruth Anne, 1967- Story of Jack Otter of Waswanipi. Cree. | DyckFehderau, Ruth Anne, 1967- Story of Jack Otter of Waswanipi. French. | Cree Board of Health and Social Services of James Bay, issuing body.

Description: Cree title romanized. | "This is a four-language translation of a single story from The Sweet Bloods of Eeyou Istchee: Stories of Diabetes and the James Bay Cree. (Sweet Bloods contains 26 stories.)" | Text in Northern East Cree, Southern East Cree, French, and English.

Identifiers: Canadiana 20200402080E | ISBN 9781989796016 (softcover)

Subjects: LCSH: Otter, Jack (Of Waswanipi)—Health. | LCSH: Diabetics—Waswanipi (First Nation)—Biography. | LCGFT: Biographies.

Classification: LCC RC660 .D92 2021 | DDC 362.1964/620092—dc23

Catalogage avant publication de Bibliothèque et Archives Canada
Titre: Chaak utir utipaachimuwin waaswaanipiihch uhchiiu = Chaak atar utipaachimuwin, waaswaanipiiuiinuu = L'histoire de Jack Otter de Waswanipi = The story of Jack Otter of Waswanipi / story by Jack Otter ; translator Northern East Cree, Luci Bobbish-Salt ; translator Southern East Cree, Louise Blacksmith ; translator French, Valérie Duro ; writer, Ruth DyckFehderau.
Autres titres: Chaak atar utipaachimuwin, waaswaanipiiuiinuu | Histoire de Jack Otter de Waswanipi | Story of Jack Otter of Waswanipi
Noms: DyckFehderau, Ruth, 1967- auteur. | DyckFehderau, Ruth Anne, 1967- Story of Jack Otter of Waswanipi. | DyckFehderau, Ruth Anne, 1967- Story of Jack Otter of Waswanipi. Cree. | DyckFehderau, Ruth Anne, 1967- Story of Jack Otter of Waswanipi. Français. | Conseil Cri de la santé et des services sociaux de la Baie-James, organisme de publication.
Description: Titre en cri romanisé. | Publiée antérieurement dans : The Sweet Bloods of Eeyou Istchee: Stories of Diabetes and the James Bay Cree. | Texte en cri de l'Est du nord, en cri de l'Est du sud, en français et en anglais.
Identifiants: Canadiana 20200402080F | ISBN 9781989796016 (couverture souple)
Vedettes-matière: RVM: Otter, Jack—Santé. | RVM: Diabétiques—Waswanipi (Première nation)—Biographies. | RVMGF: Biographies.
Classification: LCC RC660 .D92 2021 | CDD 362.1964/620092—dc23

ᐃᐦᑖᐤ ᐊᓂᑖᐦ ᓈᐹᐤ ᐧᐋᐧᓵᓂᐲ ᑯᐯᒃ, ᐹᔮᑯᓂᔮᐤ ᐅᔅᑳᑦ᙮ ᐧᐋᐱᒥᔅᑳ ᐊᓂᑖᐦ ᐋᐦ ᐱᑳᔑᒧᐧᐃᑦ ᐧᐋᐧᓵᓂᐲᐢᑎᑯᐦᒡ, ᒋᑭ ᐧᐋᐱᐦᑎᔮᒃ ᐊᓂᔫ ᔩᐲᔮᐤ ᑭᔫᐦ ᐊᓂᑎᐦ ᑳ ᐊᑯᑎᐦᑖᑦ ᐅᔅᑳᑦ ᑭᔫᐦ ᐹᐱᔮᔮᒡᐦ ᓂᒫᔅᐦ ᐋᐦ ᒫᑯᐦᒑᔮᒡ ᐦ ᑭᔫᐦ ᐋᐦ ᒌᐦ ᒋᒥᐦᑎᒥᔮᒡᐦ ᐹᔮᒄ ᐊᓂᔫ ᐅᔅᑳᑦ᙮

ᓂᒥᔫᐤ ᒫᒃ ᐆ ᑎᐹᒋᒧᐧᐃᓐ ᒑ ᑎᐹᒋᒧᓈᓂᐧᐃᒡ᙮

ᒫᐧᑳᒡ ᑳ ᐊᐧᐋᔑᔑᐅᐧᐃᑦ ᒑᒃ ᐅᑎᕽ ᐅᓃᒋᐦᐄᒄᐦ ᒌᐦ ᐧᐄᒋᒫᐤ ᐊᓂᑖᐦ ᐅᓂᑑᐦᐅᔅᒌᐧᐋᐦᒡ᙮ ᒥᒄ ᒫᒃ ᒌᐦ ᐅᑎᐦᒋᐱᔮᔮᐤ ᒑᒃ ᒑ ᒋᔅᑯᑎᒫᓱᑦ᙮ ᒫᐧᑳᒡ ᒫᒃ ᐋᐦ ᐱᒥᐱᔮᔮᒡ ᐋᐦ ᒋᔅᑯᑎᒫᓱᓈᓂᐧᐃᐧᐃᔮᒡ ᐅᑐᓯᔅᐦ ᑳ ᒌ ᐧᐄᒋᒫᑦ ᒑᒃ ᐊᓂᑖᐦ ᐧᐋᐧᓵᓂᐱᐦᒡ᙮ ᒌᐦ ᒥᒥᔨᐦᑳᑰ ᑭᔫᐦ ᑯᐃᔅᑯ ᒌᐦ ᐃᐦᑐᑖᑯ ᐊᓂᔫᐦ ᐅᑐᓯᔅᐦ ᒫᐧᑳᒡ ᐋᑳ ᐅᐦᒋ ᒌᐦ ᐧᐄᒋᒫᑦ ᐅᓃᒋᐦᐄᒄᐦ᙮ ᒥᒄ ᒫᒃ ᐊᓂᑖᐦ ᐱᑯᑎᔅᑭᒥᑳᐦᒡ ᐋᐦ ᐄᐦᑖᑦ ᐋᑯᑖᐦ ᒫᐅᒡ ᑳ ᒥᐧᔮᔮᐦᑎᐦᒃ, ᑭᔫᐦ ᐋᑯᑖᐦ ᑏᐧᐋᐦᒡ ᑳ ᒌ ᐄᔅᐱᔮᑦ ᒫᐧᑳᒡ ᐋᑳ ᒋᔅᑯᑎᒫᓱᑦ᙮ ᐊᓂᑎᐦ ᑳ ᐱᐹᐦᒡ 1980 ᒌᐦ ᑭᔅᒋᐦᐅᐧᐃᒡ ᐄᔮᔮᐅᓈᐹᔑᔑᒡ ᐹᔅᒋᓯᑭᓐᐦ ᐋᐦ ᐋᐱᒋᐦᑖᒡ, ᒌᐦ ᑭᔅᒋᐦᐆ ᑭᔫᐦ ᐧᐄᔮ ᒑᒃ, ᒥᒄ ᒫᒃ ᐋᔨᐧᐃᒄ ᑭᔫᐦ ᑳᐦ ᒋᔅᑯᑎᒫᑯᑦ ᐅᐦᑖᐧᐄᐦ ᒑ ᐋᐱᒋᐦᐋᑦ ᐊᐦᒑᐲᐦ ᑭᔫᐦ ᐊᑭᔅᑯᐦ ᑭᔫᐦ ᓯᓚᓐᑭᐧᔕᑎᔮᐤ᙮ ᒌᐦ ᐹᐱᔮᐤ ᐊᓂᑖᐦ ᐊᐧᐋᓐ ᐋᐦ ᐧᐄᐦ ᐹᒋ ᓈᓂᑑᒋᔅᒑᔮᐦᑎᐦᒃ ᐄᔮᔮᐅᐄᔮᑎᐧᐃᓂᔮᐤ, ᑳ ᒥᔅᓈᐱᔅᑭᐦᐅᑯᑦ ᐊᓂᔫᐦ ᒑᒃ, ᐊᓂᑖᐦ ᒥᓯᓂᐦᐄᑭᓂᐦᒡ ᐋᑯᑎᐦ ᑳ ᓅᑯᓯᑦ ᐊᓂᔫ ᑳ ᒥᓯᓈᐱᔅᑭᐦᐧᐋᑭᓂᐧᐃᑦ᙮ ᐊᓂᔫ ᑳ ᒥᓯᓈᐱᔅᑭᐦᐧᐋᑭᓂᐧᐃᑦ ᒫᐧᑳᒡ ᒌᐦ ᐅᐧᐋᔮᐦᐋᒻ ᒦᒋᒥᔮᐤ ᐋᐦ ᐋᐱᐧᔕᔑᔮᒡ ᐋᐦ ᐧᐄᐦ ᓂᐱᐦᑖᑦ᙮

ᐃᐦᑖᐤ ᓈᐯᐤ ᐊᓂᑌ ᐧᐋᔅᐧᐋᓂᐲᐦᒡ ᐁ ᒋᒫᔮᒡ ᐅᔅᑳᑦ, ᒑᒃ ᐁ ᐃᓯᓂᐦᑳᓱᑦ᙮ ᐧᐋᐸᒥᔅᑫ ᐊᓂᑌ ᐧᐋᔅᐧᐋᓂᐲᐤ ᔩᐲᐦᒡ ᐁ ᐹᑲᔑᒨᑦ ᒋᑲ ᐧᐋᐸᐦᑎᔮᒄ ᐊᓂᑕ ᐁ ᐧᐋᐃᓂᐦᑎᓂᔮᒡ ᐊᓂᔩ ᔩᐱᔩ ᐊᓂᑕ ᓇᐦᐋᐤ ᑳ ᐸᑲᐢᑕᐧᐁᑌᑦ ᑳ ᐅᐦᒋ ᐹᐸᔮᐦᐅᔮᒡ ᓇᒣᔅ ᐁ ᒫᒥᐦᑳᐱᑌᔮᒡ ᐁ ᒥᐦᑫᑎᔮᒡ ᒥᒍᓐ ᐁᒌ ᒋᒪᑲᐦᑕᒥᔮᒡ ᐯᔮᒄ ᐅᔅᑳᑦ᙮

ᓇᒪᔦᔩ ᒥᒄ ᐅᔩ ᑎᐹᒋᒧᐧᐃᓂᔩ ᑫ ᐧᐄᐦᑕᒄ ᐅᑕ᙮

ᒉᐧᑳᒡ ᑳ ᐅᔅᒋᓃᒎᑦ ᒑᒃ ᐊᑕᕽ, ᓅᐦᒋᒦᐦᒡ ᒌ ᐃᐦᑖᔩ ᐅᓃᒋᐦᐄᒄ᙮ ᒌ ᒋᔅᑯᑕᒫᓲ ᐧᐄᔮ ᐊᓂᑕ ᐧᐋᔅᐧᐋᓂᐲᐦᒡ, ᐅᑑᔖ ᒌ ᑲᓇᐧᐁᔮᒥᑰ᙮ ᒌ ᒥᔦᔮᐦᑖᑯᓯᔩ ᑲᔦ ᒌ ᒥᔦᔮᐦᒎ ᐊᓂᑕ ᑳ ᐃᐦᑖᑦ ᒉᐧᑳᒡ ᐁᑳ ᐅᐦᒋ ᐃᐦᑖᔮᒡ ᐅᓃᒋᐦᐄᒄ᙮ ᐅᔅᑌ ᒫᒃ ᒌ ᒥᔦᔮᐦᑕᒻ ᐊᓂᑌ ᓂᑐᐧᐄᓐ ᐁ ᐃᐦᑖᑦ ᐁᒄ ᓅᐦᒋᒦᐦᒡ ᑳᒌ ᓂᑑ ᐃᐦᑖᑦ ᒫᓐ᙮ ᐊᓂᔩᐦ ᐊᔅᒌᐤ ᐊᒋᐦᑖᓯᓐ 80 ᑳ ᐅᐦᒋ ᒋᐦᒋᐸᔮᐦᐧᑳᐤ ᐊᓂᑌ ᒫᒃ ᐃᔑ ᐯᒋ ᒌ ᓂᑑᐦᐆᒡ ᐅᔅᒋᓃᒎᒡ ᐹᔅᒋᓯᑲᓐᐦ ᐁ ᐋᐸᒋᐦᑖᐧᑖᐤ ᐁᐅᒄ ᒫᒃ ᑳ ᐃᐦᑎᑦ ᑲᔦ ᐧᐄᔮ ᒑᒃ, ᒥᒄ ᒫᒃ ᐊᑯᔅᑯᐦ ᒌ ᐋᐸᒋᐦᐁᔩᐦ ᐅᒍᐧᔖᒻ ᑲᔦ ᑳᔫᐱᔅᒋᐸᔮᒡ ᐁᐅᒄ ᒫᒃ ᐊᓂᔩᐦ ᑳ ᒋᔅᑯᑕᒫᑯᑦ ᑫᒌ ᐋᐸᒋᐦᑖᑦ ᐁ ᓂᑑᐦᐅᑦ᙮ ᐯᔮᐧᑳᐤ ᒌ ᐹᐸᔩ ᐧᐁᒥᔅᑎᑰᔫᐤ ᐊᓂᑌ ᐄᓅᔅᒌᐦᒡ ᐁ ᓈᓂᑑ ᒋᔅᑫᔮᒫᑦ ᐄᓅᐦ ᑖᓐ ᐁ ᐄᔑ ᐱᒫᑎᓯᔮᒡ ᐁᒄ ᑳ ᒪᓯᓈᐱᔅᑲᐦᐧᐋᑦ ᒑᒃ ᒌ ᓅᑯᓂᔩ ᒫᒃ ᐊᓂᔩ ᒪᓯᓈᐱᔅᑲᐦᐄᑲᓂᔩ ᒪᓯᓇᐦᐄᑲᓂᐦᒡ ᐧᐄᔮ ᐊᓐ ᓈᐯᐤ ᐁᒌ ᐅᔑᐦᑖᑦ᙮ ᒌ ᓅᑯᓲ ᒑᒃ ᐁ ᑳᐦᑲᐯᑳᐳᑦ ᑳᔫᐱᔅᒋᐸᔮᔮᒡ ᐁ ᑕᐦᑯᓇᒃ ᐁ ᐊᐱᔒᔑᔮᒡ ᐊᐧᐁᔫᔅ ᐁ ᑕᓯᐹᔅᑯᓈᑦ᙮

Dans la ville de Waswanipi, au Québec, vit un unijambiste nommé Jack. S'il vous voit nager dans la rivière Waswanipi, il vous montrera le coude de la rivière où il a un jour submergé ses jambes et où un banc de requins affamés est arrivé et reparti avec l'une d'entre elles.

Il ne s'agit pas ici de cette histoire.

Quand Jack Otter était adolescent, ses parents vivaient dans le bois. Toutefois, il devait aller à l'école et, pendant les mois d'école, il restait chez sa tante à Waswanipi. Elle était gentille et lui offrait un foyer sûr pendant les périodes où il ne pouvait pas être avec ses parents. Cependant, la vie sur le territoire était son véritable mode de vie et il allait dans le bois aussi souvent qu'il le pouvait. Comme la plupart des jeunes Cris dans les années 80, Jack pouvait chasser avec un fusil, mais son père lui avait aussi appris les méthodes traditionnelles de chasse à l'arc et aux flèches ou à la fronde. Un anthropologue passa par Eeyou Istchee un jour et prit une photo du jeune Jack, qu'il publia dans un livre. En position avec les jambes écartées, Jack y tire sur la bande d'une fronde en visant une sorte de petit gibier.

French

In the town of Waswanipi, Québec, lives a one-legged man named Jack. If he sees you swimming in the Waswanipi River, he will show you the river bend where he once submerged his legs and a school of hungry river sharks came along and nibbled one right off.

This is not that story.

When Jack Otter was a teenager, his parents lived in the bush. He had to go to school, though, and during the school months he stayed with his aunt in Waswanipi. She was kind and provided a safe home for him in the times he couldn't be with his parents. Still, living on the land was his true way of life and he went out to the bush as often as he could. Like most young Cree in the '80s, Jack could hunt with a gun, but his father had taught him the traditional ways of hunting with bow and arrow or slingshot. An anthropologist came through Eeyou Istchee once and took a photograph of the boy Jack and he published it in a book. In wide-legged stance, Jack is pulling back the band of a slingshot, aiming at some kind of small game.

English

ᐋᔥᒄ ᒌᐦ ᐊᐧᐋᔑᔒᐤ ᒑᒃ, ᐋᑯᑎᐦ ᑳ ᒋᔅᓵᔭᐦᑎᐦᒃ ᐋᐦ ᔖᑳᐅᐱᔭᑦ᙮ ᒥᒄ ᑳ ᐄᑎᑰᑦ ᐊᓂᔮᐦ ᓂᑐᐦᑯᔭᓂᔅᐧᑳᐤ ᓲᐅᑏᓯᔭᐤ ᒐ ᒦᒋᑦ ᐊ̈ᑲ ᔖᐱᒥᒋᐦᐅᑖ ᑭᔮᐦ ᒥᒄ ᒥᔑᓂᐦᐄᑭᓂᔑᔭᐤ ᒌᐦ ᒥᔭᑰ ᒐ ᐊᔭᒥᐦᑖᑦ᙮ ᐄᔑᓈᑯᓂᔭᐤ ᐊᐧᐋᓂᒌ ᐋᐦ ᔖᑳᐅᐱᔭᒡ ᑯᐃᔅᒄ ᒐ ᐄᔑ ᒦᒋᓯᒡ, ᒌᐦ ᐄᒋᔥᑖᔭᐤ, ᒥᒄ ᓂᒥ ᒥᒋᓐ ᐅᐦᒋ ᐧᐄᐦᑖᑯᓂᔭᐤ ᒑᐧᑳᔭᐤ ᐊᓂᔮ ᐋᔥᒌᐧᔖᒥᑭᓂᔭᒡ ᑯᐃᔅᒄ ᐋᐦ ᐄᔑ ᒦᒋᓯᑦ ᐊᐧᐋᓐ᙮ ᓂᒧᐃ ᓈᔥᒡ ᐅᐦᒋ ᓂᓯᑐᐦᑎᒻ ᒑᒃ ᐊᓂᔮ ᑳ ᐄᔑ ᐊᔭᒥᐦᑖᑦ᙮ ᐊᓂᔮ ᒫᒃ ᐋᐦ ᐄᔑ ᐋᔭᒧᑖᔭᒡ ᐋᐦ ᔖᑳᐅᐱᔭᓈᓂᐧᐃᐧᐃᔭᒡ, ᓂᒧᐃ ᓈᔥᒡ ᐅᐦᒋ ᓯᓵᐱᐦᐄᑯᐧᐃᒡ ᓂᑐᐦᑯᔭᓂᒡ ᑭᔮᐦ ᓂᑐᐦᑯᔭᓂᔅᐧᑳᐅᒡ ᐋᑯᑎᐦ ᑳ ᐄᑖᔭᐦᑎᐦᒃ ᐊ̈ᑲ ᓈᔥᒡ ᒫᔮᑎᓂᔭᒡ ᐋᐦ ᔖᑳᐅᐱᔭᓈᓂᐧᐃᐧᐃᔭᒡ᙮ ᓂᒧᐃ ᐅᐦᒋ ᐋᐦᑯᓯᐤ ᑭᔮᐦ ᒑᑲᑦ ᒨᔥ ᒌᐦ ᒥᔫᒥᐦᒋᐦᐆ᙮ ᓂᔮᓂᑯᑑᓐᐦ ᒥᒄ ᒌᐦ ᑖᑎᑳᔥᑖᔮᔭᐦᑎᒻ ᓈᔥᒡ ᑭᔭᐧᐹ ᐊ̈ᑲ ᐅᐦᒋ ᔖᐱᒥᒋᐦᐅᑦ= ᐋᑦ ᓈᔥᒡ ᒥᔥᒌᐦ ᒥᓂᐦᐧᑳᑦ ᓂᐲᔭᐤ ᐊ̈ᑲ ᐋᔮᐱᒡ ᐅᐦᒋ ᑖᐱᓯᒧᑦ = ᒥᒄ ᒫᒃ ᒌᐦ ᐃᐦᑎᑯᓂᔭᐤ ᒑᐧᑳᔭᐤ ᐊᑎᑎᐤ ᐋᐦ ᒋᔥᑎᒫᐧᐋᔭᐦᑎᐦᒃ᙮ ᐋᔫᐧᐃᒄ ᐋᐦ ᒥᓂᐦᐧᑳᑦ ᐋᔥᐧᑳᑎᐧᐃᔥᑖᔭᒡᐦ᙮ ᑭᔮᐦ ᒫᒃ ᒐ ᒌᐦ ᐋᐱᒋᔥᑖᑦ ᒥᒋᓂᑐᐦᑯᔭᓐᐦ ᓂᔮᓂᑯᑑᓐᐦ᙮ ᑭᔮᐦ ᒫᒃ ᒐ ᒌᐦ ᒥᓂᐦᐧᑳᑦ ᐹᔭᒄ ᑳᐲᔥᒑᐅᐲᔑᔭᒡ (ᑭᔮᐦ ᒫᒃ ᓂᔮᔪ ᑭᔮᐦ ᒫᒃ ᒥᑖᐦᑐ) ᐋᐦ ᐧᐄᒋᒥᓂᐦᐧᑳᒫᑦ ᐅᐧᐄᒑᐧᐋᑭᓐᐦ ᑳ ᒌᔑ ᒋᔅᑯᑎᒫᓯᐧᑖᐤᐦ᙮ ᒥᒄ ᐧᐋᔥ ᐹᔭᐧᑳᐤ ᒋᑭ ᓂᔮᓈᓈᐅᔕᐳᐳᐧᓈᓯᐤ ᒐ ᐄᔥᐱᔑ ᐱᒫᑎᓲᑦ᙮ ᒌᐦ ᒋᔥᑎᒫᐧᐋᔭᐦᑎᒻ ᐅᔮ ᒐ ᒌᐦ ᐃᐦᑐᑎᐦᒃ, ᒥᒄ ᐧᐋᔥ ᐹᔭᐧᑳᐤ ᒋᑭ ᐱᒫᑎᓲᐤ ᑭᔮᐦ ᒫᒃ ᒥᒄ ᐋᔥᐱᔥ ᒌᐦ ᐃᐦᑐᑎᐦᒃ ᒋᑭ ᐧᐄᐦ ᒧᒋᑭᐦᑖᐤ᙮

ᑳ ᐅᔅᒋᓃᒎᑦ ᒫᒃ ᐁᑯᑦ ᑳ ᒥᔅᑳᑲᓄᔭᒡ ᐁ ᓲᐧᐋᑲᒥᐦᐧᑫᑦ᙮ ᒌ ᐃᑎᑰ ᓂᑐᐦᑯᐄᓂᔅᐧᑫᐤ ᒉ ᒦᒋᑦ ᓲᐅᑏᓯᔫ ᐁᑳ ᓵᐸᒪᐦᒋᐦᐅᑌ ᑲᔦ ᒪᓯᓇᐦᐄᑲᓂᔑᔫ ᒌ ᒥᔭᑰ ᒉ ᐊᔭᒥᐦᑖᑦ᙮ ᐁᐅᒄ ᑳ ᐃᒋᔥᑌᔭᒡ ᐊᓂᑕ ᐊᓂᔫ ᒪᓯᓇᐦᐄᑲᓂᔫ ᐊᐧᐁᓐ ᑳ ᓲᐧᐋᑲᒥᐦᐧᑫᑦ ᐁ ᒥᔫᔅᑳᑫᒪᑲᓂᔭᒡ ᒦᒋᒥᔫ ᑫ ᒦᒋᑦ ᐁᐅᒄ ᒥᒄ ᑳ ᐃᒋᔥᑌᒡ ᓇᒧᐃ ᐅᐦᒋ ᐧᐄᐦᑖᑯᓐ ᑫᒄ ᒦᒋᒻ ᒉᔫᔅᑳᑫᒪᑲᐦᒡ᙮ ᓇᒧᐃ ᓈᔅᒡ ᐅᐦᒋ ᐊᔭᒥᐦᐄᑰ ᐅᔫ ᒑᒃ ᑫᒌ ᐅᐦᒋ ᓂᓯᑐᐦᑕᐦᒃ ᐊᓂᔫ ᐋᐦᑯᓯᐧᐃᓂᔫ᙮ ᐃᔅᑫᑳ ᓈᔅᒡ ᐅᐦᒋ ᐋᐸᑌᔭᐦᑕᒥᐦᐄᑰᒌ ᓂᑐᐦᑯᐄᓂᔅᐧᑫᐅᒡ ᑲᔦ ᓂᑐᐦᑯᐃᓂᒡ ᐁᒄ ᑳ ᐃᑌᔭᐦᑕᐦᒃ ᐁᑳ ᐧᐃᔦᔅ ᐃᑌᔭᐦᑖᑯᓂᔭᒡ᙮ ᓇᒧᐃ ᐅᐦᒋ ᒨᔑᐦᑖᐤ ᑫᒌ ᐋᐦᑯᓯᑦ ᐅᔖ ᒌ ᒥᔫᒪᐦᒋᐦᐆ ᒫᓐᐦ᙮ ᓂᔮᓂᑯᑌᐦᒡ ᑮᐹ ᒌ ᐅᔥᑖᐸᔭᐦᐄᑰ ᐊᓂᑕ ᒉᐧᑳᒡ ᐁᑳ ᓵᐸᒪᐦᒋᐦᐅᑦ ᒫᒃ ᒥᔅᑕᐦᐄ ᐁ ᒥᓂᐦᐧᑫᑦ ᓂᐱᔫ ᔮᐸᒡ ᒫᒃ ᐁ ᐹᐦᑯᑖᐦᑕᐦᒃ ᒥᒄ ᒫᒃ ᓇᒧᐃ ᔮᐸᒡ ᐅᐦᒋ ᐧᐊᓈᑌᔭᐦᑕᒥᐦᐄᑰ ᑫᐧᑳᔫ ᐁ ᐧᐄ ᐃᐦᑑᑕᐦᒃ ᐊᓂᔫ ᐅᔥᑌ ᐁ ᐃᑌᔭᐦᑕᒥᐦᐄᑯᑦ᙮ ᒌ ᐧᐄᒋᐦᐄᐧᐁᐤ ᐊᓂᑌ ᐁ ᐋᔭᒥᓯᓈᓄᔭᒡ ᐁ ᐃᔥᐧᑳᑑᔥᑌᔭᒡ᙮ ᒌ ᒪᒋᓂᑎᐦᑯᐦᐄᓲ ᑲᔦ ᐋᔥᑰ᙮ ᐁ ᒌᔑ ᒋᔅᑯᑕᒫᓯᐧᑖᐤ ᐁᒄ ᑳᒌ ᓂᑑ ᒥᓂᐦᐧᑫᐅᐱᐧᑖᐤ ᒫᓐ ᐅᐧᐄᑫᐧᐋᑲᓐ ᒥᒄ ᒋᐧᐄ ᐅᔖᒥᐸᔭᐦᑖᐤ ᒫᓐᐦ᙮ ᒥᒄ ᒫᒃ ᒥᒄ ᐯᔭᐧᑳᐤ ᓂᑲ ᔮᓈᓈᐅᔖᐳᓀᓯᓐ ᒌ ᐃᑌᔭᐦᑕᒻ᙮ ᐃᑌᔭᐦᑖᑯᓐ ᑖᐧᐯ ᓲᐦᒃ ᑫᒌ ᒨᒋᑲᐦᑖᔮᓐ ᐁᔅᒄ ᐁ ᐊᐧᐋᔒᐅᔮᓐ᙮

Quand Jack était adolescent, il apprit qu'il était diabétique. L'infirmière lui dit que cela signifiait simplement qu'il devait manger un bonbon s'il se sentait faible et lui donna une brochure. Les personnes atteintes du diabète devraient manger mieux, disait cette brochure, mais elle n'expliquait pas ce que signifiait « manger mieux ». En fait, elle ne disait qui ait vraiment un sens pour Jack. Quoi que soit le diabète, les médecins et les infirmières ne le prenaient de toute évidence pas au sérieux, donc cela ne pouvait pas être trop grave. Il ne souffrait pas et la plupart du temps, il se sentait bien. Cela pouvait parfois être gênant – il manquait d'énergie ou buvait des carafes d'eau entières sans étancher sa soif –, mais cela n'empiétait pas sur les choses plus importantes de la vie. Comme les partys de la fin de semaine. Ou un petit *buzz* de temps en temps. Ou le plaisir d'une bière fraîche (ou cinq, ou dix) après l'école avec ses amis. De toute sa vie, il n'aurait 18 ans qu'une seule fois. Il était important d'en profiter un maximum, de s'amuser autant que possible.

When Jack was a teenager, he learned that he had diabetes. The nurse said it just meant he should eat a candy if he felt weak and gave him a pamphlet. People with diabetes should eat better, it said, but it didn't explain what "eating better" meant. In fact, it didn't really say anything that made sense to Jack. Obviously, whatever diabetes was, the doctors and nurses weren't taking it seriously so it couldn't be too bad. He wasn't in pain and most of the time he felt fine. It could sometimes be inconvenient – he would run out of energy, or drink jugs of water without quenching his thirst – but it didn't interfere with more important things in life. Like parties on the weekends. Or a quick high now and then. Or the pleasure of a cold beer (or five, or ten) after school with his friends. In his whole life, he would be 18 years old only once. It was important to make the most of it, to have as much fun as he possibly could.

ᐊᓂᑖᐦ ᒌᐦ ᐄᔑ ᐋᐱᑎᓰᐤ ᒑᒃ ᐋᐦ ᓈᓈᑭᒥᐦᑖᑭᓂᐧᐃᐧᐃᔭᒡ ᐊᔅᒌᔭᐤ ᑭᔮᐦ ᓂᑐᐦᐅᐧᐃᓂᔭᐤ, ᒫᐧᑳᒡ ᒫᒃ ᐊᓂᔮ ᐋᐦ ᐄᑖᐱᑎᓰᑦ ᐋᑯᑎᐦ ᑳᐦ ᒋᔅᑯᑎᒫᓯᑦ ᒑ ᒌᐦ ᐋᐱᑎᓰᑦ ᐊᓂᑖᐦ ᐋᐦ ᓈᓈᑭᒥᐦᑖᑭᓂᐧᐃᐧᐃᔭᒡ ᓂᑑᐦᐅᐧᐃᓂᔭᐤ ᑭᔮᐦ ᑯᐃᔅᒄ ᒑ ᒌᐦ ᐃᐦᑐᑎᑭᓂᐧᐃᐧᐃᔭᒡ᙮ ᓂᔮᓂᑯᑑᓐᐦ ᒫᐧᑳᒡ ᐋᐦ ᐋᐱᑎᓰᑦ ᒋᔥᒋᑯᒡ ᑳ ᒌ ᐃᐦᑎᒃ ᐋᑳ ᔖᐱᒥᒋᐦᐅᑦ ᒑ ᒌᐦ ᐧᐄᒋᐦᐄᐧᐋᑦ ᐊᓂᑖᐦ ᐧᐃᔭᐧᐄᑎᒥᐦᒡ ᐋᐦ ᒋᔅᑯᑎᒫᓯᓈᓂᐧᐃᐧᐃᔭᒡ ᑭᔮᐦ ᓂᒧᐃ ᒨᔥ ᐅᐦᒋ ᒋᔅᒋᓰ ᒑ ᒌᐦ ᐱᐹᐃᔮᑦ ᓰᐅᑏᓯᔭᐤ᙮ ᒑᔅᒋᓯᒡ ᒫᒃ ᒥᒄ ᓇᔥᒡ ᐧᐋᔭᐱᔥᒌᔥ ᒌᐦ ᐋᐱᑎᓰᒥᑭᓂᔭᐤ ᐊᓂᔮ ᓰᐅᑏᓯᔭᐤ; ᐋᐱᐦᑎᐤ ᐋᐦ ᒌᓂᐧᑳᓂᐦᑖᔭᒡᐦ ᐲᓯᒨᐦᑳᓐᐦ ᑭᔮᐦ ᒫᒃ ᐊᑎᑎᐤ ᓈᐅᔒᔥ, (ᒑᒃ ᒦᓐ ᑳ ᒌ ᑭᐧᐃᐦᑯᔒᑦ ᐊᓂᑖᐦ ᐲᐦᒡ ᐅᑖᐹᓈᔅᑯᐦᒡ)᙮ ᑖᐹ ᐅᐦᒋ ᒋᔅᒑᔭᐦᑎᒻ ᐊᓂᔮ ᐋᐦ ᐃᐦᑎᒃ ᐋᔪᐧᐃᒄ ᐊᓂᔮ ᐋᑳ ᐹᔭᑯᓂᐦᒡ ᐅᐦᒋ ᐄᔭᔅᐱᔭᔭᒡ ᐅᔖᑳᒻ ᐅᒥᐦᑯᐦᒡ ᐅᐦᒋ ᐊᓂᔮ ᐋᐦ ᒌᐦ ᔖᑳᐅᐱᔭᑦ᙮ ᐋᑳ ᒫᒃ ᐅᐦᒋ ᒋᔅᒑᔭᐦᑎᐦᒃ ᒑᒃ ᒑᐧᑳᔭᐤ ᐊᓂᔮ ᐧᐋᐦᒋ ᐃᔭᔅᐱᔭᑦ ᒥᒄ ᑳ ᒌ ᒥᓂᐦᐧᑳᑦ, ᒥᒄ ᐋᔥᐱᔒᑦ ᑳ ᒌ ᒥᓂᐦᐧᑳᑦ ᓂᐲᔭᐤ᙮ ᐊᑎᑎᐤ ᓈᔥᒡ ᓂᒥ ᐅᐦᒋ ᒥᔪᐱᔭᔭᐤ ᐊᓂᔮ ᐅᔖᑳᒻ ᑭᔮᐦ ᒑᒃ ᐹᔭᐧᑳᐤ ᐹᔭᑯᐲᓯᒻ ᒥᒄ ᑳ ᒌ ᐄᔑ ᑭᐧᐃᐦᑯᔒᑦ ᐅᐦᒋ ᐊᓂᔮ ᓈᔥᒡ ᓃᐦᑖᐦᒡ ᐋᐦ ᐄᔅᐱᔭᔭᒡ ᐅᔖᑳᒻ ᑭᔮᐦ ᓂᑐᐦᑯᔭᓂᑭᒥᑯᐦᒡ ᑳ ᒌ ᐄᔅᐱᔭᐦᐋᑭᓂᐧᐃᑦ᙮

ᐊᓂᔮ ᒫᒃ ᒨᔥ ᐋᐦ ᒌᐦ ᐄᑐᐦᑖᑦ ᓂᑐᐦᑯᔭᓂᑭᒥᑯᐦᒡ ᒑᒃ ᒥᓯᐧᐋ ᐊᐧᐋᔭᐤᐦ ᑳ ᒋᔅᒑᔭᒥᑯᑦ᙮ ᑳ ᒌ ᐄᑎᑯᑦ, “ᑭᒋᒥᐧᔮᔭᐦᑖᓈᔥᑎᑳ ᐅᑎᐦ ᒑᒃ, ᐋᐧᐄᒋᒑ ᐊᓐ ᓈᔥᒡ ᐋᐦ ᐧᐄᐦᑭᐦᒡ ᐅᑎᐦ ᒦᒋᒻ, ᑭᔮᐦ ᒫᒃ ᐋᐦ ᒥᐧᔮᒡᐦ ᐅᑎᐦ ᓂᐹᐧᐃᓐᐦ, ᑭᔮᐦ ᒫᒃ ᓇᔥᒡ ᐋᐦ ᒥᒥᔪᔑᒡ ᐅᑎᐦ ᓂᑐᐦᑯᔭᓂᔅᐧᑳᐅᒡ᙮”

ᑫᒃ ᒌ ᐊᔮᐤ ᐋᐸᑎᓯᐧᐃᓂᔫ ᐁ ᓇᓈᑲᒋᐦᑖᑦ ᐁ ᓂᑑᐦᐅᓈᓄᔭᒡ ᒥᒄ ᒫᒃ ᐁᑎᑑ ᒌᐧᐄ ᒋᔅᑫᔭᐦᑕᒻ ᐅᔫ ᐋᐸᑎᓯᐧᐃᓂᔫ ᐁᒄ ᑳ ᒋᔅᑯᑕᒫᓯᑦ᙮ ᒌ ᐋᐸᑎᓰ ᐁᔫ ᒌ ᒋᔅᑯᑕᒫᓰ᙮ ᐋᔥᑰ ᒫᒃ ᐊᓂᑌ ᐁ ᐋᐸᑎᓯᑦ ᓇᒧᐃ ᐅᐦᒋ ᐧᐄᐦ ᓵᐸᒪᐦᒋᐦᐆ ᐁᒄ ᓇᒧᐃ ᐅᐦᒌ ᐧᐄᒐᐸᑎᓰᒣᐤ ᐊᓂᔫᐦ ᑳ ᓅᑖᐦᑎᐧᑫᔭᐧᑖᐤ, ᑲᔦ ᒌ ᐧᐊᓐᒋᔅᒋᓰ ᒫᓐᐦ ᑫᒌ ᐊᔮᑦ ᓰᐅᑏᔅ᙮ ᑫᔅᒋᓯᒡ ᑮᐹ, ᒌ ᒦᒎ ᒥᒄ ᓇᒧᐃ ᒋᓀᐅᔥ ᐅᐦᒋ ᐧᐄᒋᐦᐄᑯ, ᐧᐃᔦᔅ ᐋᐱᐦᑑ ᑎᐸᐦᐄᑲᓐ ᒫᒃ ᐅᔥᑌᔒᔥ, ᐁᒄ ᒦᓐ ᑳ ᐃᔅᐸᔮᐦᑦ ᐊᓂᔫ ᑲᒌ ᐃᔅᐸᔮᐦᑦ ᐁ ᒋᐦᒋ ᐋᐸᑎᓯᒡ (ᒌ ᓂᐹᐤ ᐅᑖᐹᓂᐦᒡ)᙮ ᓇᒧᐃ ᐅᐦᒋ ᒋᔅᑫᔭᐦᑕᒻ ᐅᒥᐦᒄ ᐊᓂᔫ ᑳ ᐃᐦᑑᑖᑯᑦ ᐁ ᔖᑳᐅᐸᔭᔭᒡ ᐊᓂᔫᐦ ᐅᐦᒋ ᐁ ᒎᐧᐋᑲᒥᐦᐧᑫᑦ ᐁ ᐃᑖᔅᐱᓀᑦ᙮ ᐁᐅᒄ ᐊᓂᔫ ᑳ ᐃᐦᑑᑖᑯᑦ ᐁᑳ ᓵᐸᒪᐦᒋᐦᐅᑦ ᐁ ᐃᔅᐧᑳᐦᒋᐸᔭᓂᔭᒡ ᐅᔖᑳᒻ᙮ ᓈᔅᒡ ᒫᒃ ᒌᐧᐄ ᓯᔅᑲᒋᐦᐄᑰ ᐅᔫ ᐁ ᐃᔅᐸᔭᑦ ᒌᐧᐄ ᓈᓂᑑᐧᐁᔭᐦᑕᒻ ᑖᓐ ᑫᒌ ᐃᔑ ᐧᐄᒋᐦᐄᓯᑦ ᒥᒄ ᒫᒃ ᓇᒧᐃ ᐅᐦᒋ ᒋᔅᑫᔭᐦᑕᒻ ᑖᓐ ᑫᒌ ᐃᐦᑎᑦ᙮ ᐁᒄ ᐋᐦᒡ ᑳ ᒥᓂᐦᐧᑫᑦ ᐃᔅᑯᑌᐧᐋᐳᔫ᙮ ᐁᒄ ᐋᐦᒡ ᓇᒧᐃ ᐅᐦᒋ ᒋᐦᑳᐧᐋᒋᐸᔭᓂᔫ ᐅᔖᑳᒻ ᐁᑳ ᐯᔭᑯᓂᐦᒡ ᐅᐦᒋ ᐃᐦᑕᑯᓂᔭᒡ ᐁᒄ ᑫᒃ ᒌ ᐃᔅᐸᔫ ᒣᔑᑯᒻ ᐲᓯᒻ ᐯᔭᐧᑳᐤ ᐁ ᐋᐧᑫᔭᐦᑕᐦᒃ ᐊᓂᔫᐦ ᐅᐦᒋ ᐁ ᒥᔅᑕ ᐃᔅᐧᑳᐦᒋᐸᔭᓂᔭᒡ ᐅᔖᑳᒻ ᐋᐦᑯᓯᐅᑲᒥᑯᐦᒡ ᒫᒃ ᒌ ᐃᔅᐸᔮᐦᐋᑲᓅ ᑕᐦᐧᑖᐤ ᐅᔫ ᐁ ᐃᔅᐸᔭᑦ᙮

ᒥᓯᐧᐁ ᐋᐸᑎᓰᓯᐦ ᐊᓂᑌ ᐊᐦᑯᓯᐅᑲᒥᑯᐦᒡ ᑫᒃ ᒌ ᓂᓯᑑᓈᑰ᙮ “ᓅᐧᐊᒡ ᒋ ᒥᔦᔭᐦᑌᓈᑫ ᐅᑕ ᐁ ᐃᐦᑖᔭᓐ, ᒑᒃ,” ᒌᔑ ᓈᓈᑕᐦᑯᒥᑰ᙮ “ᐁᐅᒄ ᔮᑦ ᓂᒦᒋᒥᓈᓐ ᓈᔅᒡ ᐁ ᐧᐄᐦᑲᐦᒡ ᐧᐁᐦᒋ ᑕᑯᔑᓂᔭᓐ᙮ ᓇᒧᐃ ᐋ ᑲᔦ ᐊᓂᒌ ᓂᑐᐦᑯᐄᓂᔅᐧᑫᔅᒡ ᑳ ᐃᐦᑑᑖᔅᐧᑳᐤ ᓈᔅᒡ ᐁ ᒥᔦᔑᐧᑖᐤ᙮”

Jack devint agent de conservation et, en parallèle, il poursuivait ses études pour devenir garde-chasse. Parfois, au travail, il se sentait soudain bien trop faible pour faire le travail que font les forestiers et il ne se souvenait pas toujours d'avoir un bonbon sur lui. Lorsqu'il s'en souvenait, le bonbon ne fonctionnait que peu de temps; au bout d'une demi-heure environ, il finissait là où il avait commencé (endormi dans le camion). Il ne le savait pas, mais sa soudaine faiblesse provenait d'un taux de sucre erratique dans le sang causé par le diabète. Frustré et voulant échapper à ce cycle, mais sans savoir comment, Jack commença à boire plus qu'auparavant. Son taux de sucre devint encore plus irrégulier et, une fois par mois environ, il tombait dans un coma diabétique ou hypoglycémique et quelqu'un devait l'emmener à l'hôpital.

Jack became a conservation officer and, on the side, he studied further to be a game warden. Sometimes at work he suddenly felt much too weak to do the work forestry guys do, and he didn't always remember to carry a piece of candy. When he did remember, the candy worked only a short time; after a half hour or so, he would be right back where he started (asleep in the truck). He didn't know it, but his sudden weakness came from erratic blood sugar levels caused by diabetes. Frustrated and wanting to escape the cycle but not knowing how, Jack began to drink more than before. His sugar levels became even more erratic, and once a month or so he collapsed into a diabetic or hypoglycemic coma and someone would have to take him to the hospital.

Les gens de l'hôpital le reconnaissaient tous. « Tu dois vraiment aimer cet endroit, Jack, plaisantaient-ils. Ce doit être à cause de notre délicieuse nourriture d'hôpital ou de nos lits confortables, ou peut-être de nos jolies infirmières ».

The people at the hospital all recognized him. "You must really love it here, Jack," they would joke. "It must be our tasty hospital food. Or comfortable beds. Or maybe it's our cute nurses."

ᓂᒧᐃ ᓇᔥᒡ ᒥᐦᒑᑐᒌᔑᑳᐤᐦ ᔖᔥ ᒦᓐ ᑭᑎ ᐋᐱᑎᓰᐤ ᐋᐦ ᑎᐦᑯᓂᐦᒃ ᓂᑐᐦᑯᔨᓐᐦ ᑭᔮᐦ ᐄᓐᓯᑕᓐ᙮

ᒥᓯᐧᐋ ᒌᐦ ᒋᔅᒑᔨᐦᑎᒧᒡ ᐊᓂᑖᐦ ᐋᐦ ᒥᔥᑎᑯᔅᑳᔨᒡ ᐋᐦ ᐋᐦᐱᑎᓰᒡ ᒑ ᑳᔥᒋᐱᑖᔮᔥᑯᔑᐦᒡ ᑭᔮᐦ ᒑ ᒫᑯᒥᑯᒡ ᒥᓂᑐᔥᐦ᙮ ᓂᒧᐃ ᒫᒃ ᓈᔥᒡ ᐅᐦᒋ ᐃᔮᐱᑖᔨᐦᑎᒧᒡ ᐅᔮ᙮ ᒑᒃ ᑳ ᒥᐦᑖᔨᐦᑎᐦᒃ ᓈᔥᒡ ᓈᐅᔥ ᐋᑳ ᒥᐧᔮᔨᒡ ᐊᓂᔮᐦ ᐧᐄᔨ ᐋᐦ ᒌᐦ ᑳᔥᒋᐱᑖᔮᔥᑯᔑᐦᒃ ᐋᐦ ᐃᐦᑎᔨᒡᐦ ᐊᓂᔮᐦ ᐅᐧᐄᒑᐧᐋᑭᓐᐦ, ᐊᓂᔮᐦ ᐅᐧᐄᒑᐧᐋᑭᓐᐦ ᒥᒄ ᐧᐋᔨᐱᔥᒌᔥ ᔖᔥ ᒥᐧᔮᔨᐤᐦ ᐋᑯᐦ ᐧᐄᔨ ᒑᒃ ᒥᐦᒑᑐᑎᐧᐃᔥᑖᐤᐦ ᓂᒥ ᐅᐦᒋ ᒥᐧᔮᔨᐤᐦ᙮ ᐋᑦ ᒥᒄ ᓈᔥᒡ ᐊᐱᔒᔥ ᐧᐃᔮᓯᓈᑯᓯᑦ ᐅᔑᑳᐦᒡ ᐧᐋᔥ ᐧᐄᐱᒡ ᒌᐦ ᒫᔮᑎᓂᔨᐤ᙮ ᐋᑎ ᐅᑖᑯᔑᔨᒡᐦ, ᐆᓈᐱᑎᓰᒡᐦ, ᐊᓂᔮᐦ ᐅᑎᐦᒌᐦ ᑭᔮᐦ ᐅᓯᑦᐦ ᓈᔥᒡ ᐋᐦ ᒌᐦ ᐱᐹᑭᓂᔨᒡᐦ᙮ ᐋᔪᐧᐃᒄ ᑭᔮᐦ ᑳ ᐃᐦᑎᒃ ᓈᓈᓂᒌᒻ ᐋᑳ ᐧᐋᐱᐦᑎᐦᒃ᙮ ᒑᒃ ᒫᒃ ᒌᐦ ᐄᔑᓈᑯᓂᔨᐤ ᒑ ᐧᐃᔮᔥᑐᑎᑭᓂᐧᐃᐧᐃᔨᒡᐦ ᐊᓂᔮ ᐅᔥᒌᔑᒄᐦ ᑳ ᐄᔥᐱᔥ ᐋᑳ ᐧᐋᐱᐦᑎᐦᒃ, ᐊᓂᑎᐦ ᑭᔨᐧᐹ ᒑ ᒌᐦ ᐅᐦᒋ ᐃᐦᑐᑎᐦᒃ ᑯᐃᔅᒄ ᐅᑖᐱᑎᓰᐧᐃᓐ᙮ ᓈᔥᒡ ᐋᐦ ᒌᐦ ᒥᒫᐦᒌᔨᐦᑎᒃ ᐅᐦᒋ ᐊᓂᔮ ᐋᑳ ᐅᐦᒋ ᒥᔪᐱᒫᑎᓰᑦ᙮ ᓂᒧᐃ ᑭᔨᐧᐹ ᓈᔥᒡ ᐋᐦᐧᑳᒡ ᐅᐦᒋ ᐃᐦᑎᐤ, ᒥᒄ ᓈᔥᒡ ᐋᐦ ᒌᐦ ᐲᒋᔥᑳᒋᐦᐄᑯᑦ ᐊᓂᔮ ᐋᐦ ᐃᐦᑎᒃ᙮ ᑭᒫ ᐃᐦᑎᑯᐦᒡ ᐊᓂᑖᐦ ᒑ ᒌᐦ ᐃᐦᑎᔮᓐ, ᑳ ᒌ ᐄᑖᔨᐦᑎᐦᒃ, ᐊᑎᑎᐤ ᒑ ᒌᐦ ᒥᔪᐱᒫᑎᓯᔮᓐ᙮

ᐊᓂᔮ ᑳ ᐱᐳᓂᔨᒡ 2004 ᑳ ᐄᒋᔥᑖᔨᒡ, ᐊᓂᑖᐦ ᓲᑎᐧᓵᓐ ᐋᑯᑖᐦ ᑳᐦ ᐋᐱᑎᓰᑦ ᒑᒃ, ᐋᐦ ᓈᑭᑎᐧᐋᔨᐦᑎᑭᓂᐧᐃᐧᐃᔨᒡ ᐊᔅᒌᔨᐤ ᑭᔮᐦ ᓂᑐᐦᐅᐧᐃᓂᔨᐤ᙮ ᑳ ᐧᐄᒑᐧᐋᑦ ᐊᓂᔮ ᐹᔨᒄ ᐅᐧᐄᒑᐧᐋᑭᓐᐦ ᐋᐦ ᒫᑎᐧᐊᓂᐧᐃᐧᐃᔨᒡ ᐊᓂᑖᐦ

ᑳ ᒥᔮᑲᓅᒡ ᑮᐹ ᐅᓂᑎᐦᑯᐄᓂᒻᐦ ᑲᔦ ᐅᓂᑐᐦᑯᐄᓈᐴᓐ ᐁᒄ ᑳ ᒥᔫᐸᔨᑦ ᒦᓐ ᒉᒌ ᓂᑑ ᐋᐸᑎᓯᑦ᙮

ᒌ ᒋᔅᒉᔨᐦᑕᒥᔫ ᐊᓂᔫ ᓅᐦᑖᑕᐧᑫᓰᐦ ᑳ ᐧᐄᒑᐸᑎᓰᒫᑦ ᒉᒌ ᐃᔅᐸᔨᑦ ᐊᐧᐁᓐ ᐅᔫ ᐁ ᐄᑖᐸᑎᓯᑦ ᒉᒌ ᑳᔅᑲᐦᐆᑯᑦ ᐧᐊᑎᐦᑯᓂᔫ ᒫᒃ ᓯᒋᒣᐤᐦ ᒉᒌ ᒪᒫᑯᒥᑯᑦ᙮ ᓇᒧᐃ ᒫᒃ ᓈᔅᒡ ᐅᐦᒋ ᒪᒫᒥᑐᓀᔨᐦᑕᒥᐦᐄᑰᒡ ᐅᔫ᙮ ᒑᒃ ᒫᒃ ᒉᒃ ᒌ ᐧᐋᐸᐦᑕᒻ ᐁᑳ ᓴᒫᒡ ᒥᐧᔮᔨᒡ ᐊᓂᑕ ᐁᒌ ᑳᔅᑲᐦᐆᑯᑦ ᒥᔅᑎᒄ ᐁᒄ ᐊᓂᔫᐦ ᐅᐧᐄᒉᐧᐋᑲᓐᐦ ᓈᔅᒡ ᐧᐄᐸᒡ ᐁᒌ ᒥᐧᔮᔨᒡ᙮ ᐋᑦ ᐊᓂᑕ ᒥᒄ ᐊᐱᔒᔥ ᐁᒌ ᑳᔅᑲᔑᓂᑦ ᐁᑳ ᒦᐦᐧᑲᒡ ᓅᑯᓂᔨᒡ ᒉᒃ ᒌ ᒥᔫᐸᔨᓂᔫ᙮ ᐃᔅᑯᑕᒃ ᒫᒃ ᑳᔖᐸᑎᓯᒡ ᐧᐁᑖᑯᔑᔨᒡ ᑳᐦ ᒌᐧᐁᒡ ᒌ ᐹᒋᐸᔨᓂᔫᐦ ᐅᑎᐦᒌᐦ ᑲᔦ ᐅᓯᑦᐦ᙮ ᑲᔦ ᒉᒃ ᓇᒧᐃ ᐅᐦᒋ ᐃᔥᐱᔥ ᓇᐦᐋᐴ᙮ ᒉᒃ ᒥᒄ ᐁ ᐴᐧᐊᓈᑯᐦᒡ ᐁ ᐃᔑᓇᐦᒃ ᒉᐧᑳᔫ ᐁᒄ ᑳ ᓂᑐᐧᐁᔨᐦᑖᑯᓂᔨᒡ ᒉᒌ ᒫᒋᓯᑲᓄᔨᐧᑳᐤ ᐅᔅᒌᔑᒄ ᔮᒄ ᒦᓐ ᒉᒌ ᓂᑑ ᐋᐸᑎᓯᑦ᙮ ᓈᔅᒡ ᓇᓈᐦᑰ ᐁᒌ ᐃᔅᐸᔨᑦ ᐁᑳ ᒥᔫᐱᒫᑎᓰᑦ᙮ ᑖᐧᐯᐦ ᑮᐸ ᒧᔮᒻ ᐁᑳ ᓈᔅᒡ ᐋᐸᑌᔨᐦᑖᑯᓂᔨᒡ ᑖᓐ ᑳ ᐊᐃᐦᑖᔅᐱᓀᑦ ᒥᒄ ᐁᐅᒄ ᑳ ᐃᐦᑑᑖᑯᑦ ᓈᔅᒡ ᒌᐧᐄ ᓴᔅᑲᒋᐦᐄᑰ᙮ ᑲᒫ ᐃᐦᑕᑯᐦᒡ ᑖᓐ ᒉᒌᔑ ᐧᐄᒋᐦᐄᑯᔮᓐ, ᐁ ᐃᑌᔨᐦᑕᒃ᙮

2004 ᑳ ᐃᒋᔥᑌᒡ ᐊᔅᒌᐤ ᐊᒋᐦᑖᓯᓐ ᓲᑎᐧᓵᓐ ᒌ ᐋᐸᑎᓰ ᒑᒃ ᑳ ᓇᓈᑲᒋᐦᑖᑦ ᐁ ᓂᑑᐦᐅᓈᓄᔨᒡ ᑲᔦ ᐁ ᐅᒋᐧᑳᒑᓄᔨᒡ᙮ ᒌ ᐃᐦᑖᔫᐦ ᐯᔭᒄ ᐅᐧᐄᒉᐧᐋᑲᓐ ᐁᒌ ᐧᐄᒉᐧᐋᑦ ᔮᒡ ᐧᑖᔅ ᐁᒌ ᐃᔅᐸᔨᔨᒡ ᒉᒃ ᐧᐁᓵᒻ ᒌᓂᐧᐋᓂᐸᔨᔨᒡ ᐊᓂᔫ

Quelques jours plus tard, en possession de pilules ou d'insuline, il reprenait le travail.

A few days later, with pills or insulin in hand, he'd be back at work again.

Tous les gars au travail savaient que les travaux forestiers impliquent de se faire griffer par des branches et des insectes. Personne ne s'en plaignait vraiment. Jack commença à remarquer que ses griffures mettaient des semaines à guérir, mais que celles de ses amis guérissaient, comme d'habitude, en quelques jours. Des égratignures peu profondes, à peine visibles sur la peau de Jack, commencèrent à s'infecter. À la fin de la journée, quand il rentrait du travail, ses mains et ses pieds étaient enflés. Il avait également du mal à bien voir. Finalement, sa vision devint si trouble qu'il dut subir une opération au laser seulement pour pouvoir faire son travail. Tellement de problèmes de santé. Bien sûr, ils semblaient tous mineurs, mais ils commençaient à être gênants. Si seulement il pouvait y faire quelque chose.

All the guys at work knew that forestry jobs involve getting scratched up by branches and insects. No one really complained about it. Jack began to notice that his scratches took weeks to heal but his friends' scratches healed in a few days as usual. Shallow scrapes that barely showed up on Jack's skin began to infect. At the end of the day, when he came home from work, his hands and feet were swollen. He was having a hard time seeing clearly too. Eventually, his vision got so cloudy that he needed laser eye surgery just to be able to do his work. So many health problems. Sure, they all seemed minor, but they were getting to be annoying. If only there were something he could do.

En 2004, Jack travaillait comme agent de conservation à Radisson. Un ami et lui assistaient à un tournoi de golf à Val d'Or et reconduisaient la voiturette de golf à son stationnement lorsqu'ils virent

In 2004, Jack was working as a conservation officer in Radisson. He and a friend attended a golf benefit in Val D'Or and were returning the golf cart to its parking place when they saw something

ᐹᐤᓪ ᐧᑖᕐ ᐧᑳᓪᑉ ᐋᐦ ᐧᐄᐦ ᐅᔑᐦᐋᑭᓂᐧᐃᐧᐃᔨᒡᐦ ᔓᐧᐃᔮᓐᐦ ᐊᓂᔮᐦ ᒫᒃ ᐊᓂᑖᐦ ᑳ ᐄᔑ ᒌᐧᐋᐱᔨᐦᐋᒡ ᐊᓂᔮᐦ ᐅᒑᐹᓈᔥᑯᔥ ᑳ ᐋᐱᒋᐦᐋᒡ ᑳ ᐧᐋᐱᐦᑎᐦᒡ ᒑᐧᑳᔨᐤ ᐊᓂᑖᐦ ᒫᔅᑭᓈᐦᒡ ᐋᐦ ᒋᐱᔥᑖᔨᒡ᙮ ᐊᓂᑖᐦ ᑳ ᐄᔑ ᐧᐋᔪᐱᔨᔨᒡᐦ ᐊᓂᔮᐦ ᐅᐧᐄᒑᐧᐋᑭᓐᐦ ᐋᑳ ᐅᐦᒋ ᐧᐄᐦ ᐱᔥᑎᐦᐋᒥᔨᒡᐦ, ᓈᔥᒡ ᓲᐦᒡ ᐋᐦ ᒌᐦ ᐧᐋᔪᐱᔨᔨᒡ = ᐧᐋᓵ ᒋᔥᒋᑯᒡ᙮ ᑳ ᐧᑳᑎᐱᔑᐦᒡ ᑭᔮᐦ ᓈᐦᐋᐤ ᐊᓂᑎᐦ ᐅᔅᑳᑎᐦᒡ ᒑᒃ ᐋᑯᑎᐦ ᑳᐦ ᑎᐦᑭᐦᐅᑯᑦ ᐊᓂᔮᐦ ᐅᒑᐹᓈᔥᑯᔥ᙮

ᐊᓂᔮᐦ ᒑᒃ ᐅᐧᐄᒑᐧᐋᑭᓐᐦ ᑳ ᐧᐃᓂᔥᑳᔨᒡᐦ ᑭᔮᐦ ᑳ ᐧᑳᑎᐱᓈᔨᒡᐦ ᐊᓂᔮᐦ ᐅᒑᐹᔥᑯᔥᐦ ᑭᔮᐦ ᑳ ᐧᐄᒋᐦᐋᑦ ᒑᒃᐦ ᐋᐦ ᓃᐳᐧᐃᔨᒡᐦ᙮ ᒥᒄ ᒫᒃ ᓂᒥ ᒌᔨᐧᐊ ᐅᐦᒋ ᒌᐦ ᓃᐳ ᒑᒃ, ᐋᐦ ᒌᐦ ᓈᐧᑖᐱᔨᔨᒡ ᐊᓂᔮ ᐅᔅᑳᑦ᙮ ᐊᓂᑖᐦ ᐁᐃᒥᔅ ᓂᑐᐦᑯᔨᓂᑭᒥᑯᐦᒡ ᐋᑯᑖᐦ ᑳ ᐄᔅᐱᔨᐦᐄᑯᑦ ᐊᓂᔮᐦ ᐅᐧᐄᒑᐧᐋᑭᓐᐦ, ᐊᓯᓃᐦ ᑳ ᒋᑭᒧᐦᐋᑭᓂᐧᐃᐧᐃᔨᒡᐦ ᑭᔮᐦ ᑳᐦ ᒥᔮᑭᓂᐧᐃᑦ ᓂᑐᐦᑯᔨᓂᔨᐤ ᒐ ᐧᐄᒋᐦᐄᑯᑦ᙮ ᐊᓂᑖᐦ ᐧᐋᐧᓵᓂᐲ ᐋᑯᑖᐦ ᑳ ᐄᔑ ᒌᐧᐋᒋᔑᐦᐧᐋᑭᓂᐧᐃᑦ ᐹᑎᔥ ᒋᔥᒋᐧᐊ ᒌᐦ ᒦᓂᐧᐋᑎᓰᒑ᙮

ᑳᐦ ᐋᐦᑯᓯᑦ ᐊᓂᔮ ᐅᔅᑳᑦ᙮ ᓈᔥᒡ ᐋᐦ ᒌᐦ ᐋᐦᑯᓯᑦ᙮ ᑳ ᒌ ᑯᔥᑯᐱᔨᑦ ᐋᐦ ᑎᐱᔅᑳᔨᐤ ᐋᐦ ᐧᐄᐦ ᐹᑯᒧᐧᐃᒥᒋᐦᐅᑦ ᑭᔮᐦ ᐊᔥᑭᓂᒌᔑᑳᐤᐦ ᓈᔥᒡ ᐋᑳ ᐅᐦᒋ ᔔᐱᒥᒋᐦᐅᑦ ᑭᔮᐦ ᐋᐦ ᓈᓈᒥᐱᔨᑦ᙮ ᐃᔮᒄ ᓈᔥᑎᔨᒡ ᑳ ᓈᐧᑖᐱᔨᔨᒡ ᐅᔅᑭᓐ, ᒥᒄ ᑳ ᐄᑖᔨᐦᑎᐦᒃ ᐋᑯᑖᐦ ᐃᐦᑏᑭᒑ ᐊᐧᐋᓐ ᐋᐦ ᓈᐧᑖᐱᔨᔨᒡ ᐅᔅᑭᓐ᙮ ᒑᒃ ᑳ ᐄᑐᐦᑖᑦ ᓂᑐᐦᑯᔨᓂᑭᒥᑯᐦᒡ ᐋᐦ ᒌᐦ ᓂᑎᐧᐋᔨᐦᑎᐦᒃ ᓂᑐᐦᑯᔨᓂᔨᐤ ᒐ ᐧᐄᒋᐦᐄᑯᑦ ᐊᓂᔮᐦ ᒨᔥ ᐋᐦ

ᐅᒑᐹᓂᔑᔫ ᑳ ᐱᒥᐸᔨᐦᑖᔨᒡ᙮ ᑳ ᐧᑫᑎᐸᔨᔨᒡ ᑳ ᓇᐸᑲᐦᐆᑌᔨᐦᒡ ᐊᓂᔫ ᐅᔅᑳᑦ ᒑᒃ᙮

ᑳ ᐧᐄᐧᐄᔨᒡ ᐊᓂᔫ ᐅᐧᐄᑫᐧᐋᑲᓐ ᒑᒃ ᑳ ᑯᐃᔅᑯᐱᑕᒥᔨᒡ ᐊᓂᔫ ᐅᒑᐹᓂᔑᔫ ᐁᒄ ᑳᐧᐄ ᐧᐄᒋᐦᐄᑯᑦ ᐁ ᐱᔑᑰᑦ᙮ ᓇᒧᐃ ᒫᒃ ᐅᐦᒌ ᐱᒧᐦᑌᐤ᙮ ᐯᔮᒄ ᐊᓂᔫ ᐅᔅᑳᒡ ᒌ ᓈᐧᑖᐦᐅᑌᔫ ᐊᓂᔫ ᑳ ᐧᑫᑕᐱᔑᓂᐧᑖᐤ᙮ ᐋᐦᑯᓰᐅᑲᒥᑯᐦᒡ ᒫᒃ ᒌ ᐃᔅᐸᔨᐦᐄᑰ ᐊᓂᔫ ᐅᐧᐄᑫᐧᐋᑲᓐᐦ ᐊᓂᑌ ᐁᐃᒧᔅ ᒌ ᐃᔅᐸᔨᐦᐄᑰ ᐊᓂᑌ ᑳ ᑖᐱᐦᑕᑖᑲᓄᔨᒡ ᐊᓂᔫ ᐅᔅᑳᑎᑲᓐ ᑲᔦ ᒌ ᐊᓯᓃᐦᑳᓂᐦᑲᐦᑖᑲᓅᔫ᙮ ᒌ ᒦᔭᑲᓅ ᑲᔦ ᓂᑐᐦᑯᐃᓐᐦ ᐁᑳ ᑫᒌ ᒨᔑᐦᑖᑦ ᐊᓂᔫ ᐅᔅᑳᑦ ᐁᒄ ᑳᐤ ᑳ ᒌᐧᐁᑦ ᐊᓂᑌ ᐧᐋᔅᐧᐋᓂᐲᐦᒡ ᑫ ᐊᔓᐧᐋᐸᐦᑕᐦᒃ ᐊᓂᔫ ᐅᔅᑳᑦ ᑫᒌ ᒥᐧᔮᔨᒡ᙮

ᒌ ᒨᔑᐦᑖᐤ ᐁ ᐋᐦᑯᓯᑦ ᐊᓂᔫ ᐅᔅᑳᒡ᙮ ᓈᔅᒡ ᒌ ᐋᐦᑯᓰ᙮ ᓂᔮᓂᑯᑌᐦᒡ ᒌ ᐯᑯᐦᐄᑰ ᐁ ᑎᐱᔅᑳᔨᒡ ᐁᐧᐄ ᐹᑯᒧᑦ ᐁ ᐃᑕᒪᐦᒋᐦᐅᑦ, ᑲᔦ ᐃᔅᑲᓂᒌᔑᑳᐤ ᓇᒧᐃ ᐅᐦᒋ ᔖᐸᒪᐦᒋᐦᐆ ᑲᔦ ᒌ ᓇᓇᒥᐸᔫ᙮ ᐁᒄ ᑮᐹ ᔮᒄ ᑳ ᓈᐧᑖᐦᑕᑖᑦ ᐅᔅᑲᓐ; ᓈᓂᑑ ᐁᑯᓐ ᐃᑕᒪᐦᒋᐦᐅᔨᑫ ᒥᓯᐧᐁ ᐊᐧᐁᓐ ᐁᒌ ᓈᐧᑖᐦᑕᑖᑦ ᐅᔅᑲᓐ᙮ ᔮᐸᒡ ᒫᒃ ᒌ ᐃᑐᐦᑌᐤ ᓂᑐᐦᑯᐃᓂᑲᒥᑯᐦᒡ ᐁ ᓂᑐᐧᐁᔨᐦᑕᐦᒃ ᑫᒌ ᒦᔭᑲᓅᑦ ᓂᑐᐦᑯᐃᓂᔫ ᐁᑳ ᑫᒌ

quelque chose juste devant eux sur la route. L'ami de Jack tourna violemment le volant pour l'éviter et la voiturette fit une embardée un peu trop brusque. Elle se retourna et atterrit en partie sur la jambe à l'envers de Jack.

just ahead on the road. Jack's friend swung the driver's wheel to avoid it, and the cart swerved – a little too much. It flipped right over and landed partly on Jack's upside-down leg.

L'ami de Jack sortit, repoussa la voiturette à la verticale et aida Jack à se relever. Jack ne pouvait cependant pas se tenir sur sa jambe. Elle avait été cassée dans l'accident. Son ami l'emmena à l'hôpital d'Amos où le médecin réduisit sa fracture et lui plâtra la jambe. Il lui donna quelque chose contre la douleur et Jack rentra chez lui à Waswanipi pour y guérir.

Jack's friend got out and pushed the cart upright again and helped Jack to his feet. But Jack couldn't stand on his leg. It had broken in the accident. His friend took him to the Amos hospital where the doctor set the leg and casted it, gave him something for pain, and Jack went home to Waswanipi to heal.

Sa jambe le faisait souffrir. Elle le faisait beaucoup souffrir. Parfois, Jack se réveillait la nuit avec des envies de vomir et, toute la journée, il se sentait faible et tremblant. C'était la première fois qu'il avait un os cassé; il est probable que tous les os cassés en voie de guérison causaient les mêmes sensations. Jack alla toutefois à la clinique et demanda

The leg hurt. It really hurt. Sometimes Jack would wake in the night wanting to vomit, and all day long he felt weak and shaky. It was his first broken bone; probably all healing broken bones felt like this. Still, Jack went to the clinic and asked for a pill to control the nausea and weakness while his leg healed. The doctor eyed him strangely. The pain should have

ᒌᐦ ᐧᐄᐦ ᐹᑯᒧᐧᐃᒥᒋᐦᐅᑦ ᑭᔮᐦ ᐊᓂᔮ ᐋᑳ ᔖᐱᒥᒋᐦᐅᑦ ᐅᐦᒋ ᐊᓂᔮ ᐅᔅᑳᑦ᙮ ᓈᔥᒡ ᐋᐦ ᑯᔥᐧᑳᐱᒥᑯᑦ ᐊᓂᔮᐦ ᓂᑐᐦᑯᔨᓐᐦ᙮ ᐊᐧᑳᑎᑯᑦ, “ᔕᔥ ᐧᐋᔥ ᐊᑐᒡ ᒋᒧᔑᐦᑖᓐ ᐋᐦ ᐋᐦᑯᓯᔨᓐ ᐊᓐ ᒋᔅᑳᑦ, ᑖᐹ ᐃᐦᑎᐤ ᐊᐧᐋᓐ ᐋᐦ ᒌᐦ ᓈᐧᑖᐱᔨᔨᒡ ᐅᔅᑭᓐ,” ᐄᑎᑰ᙮ ᒫᓂᐧᔖᔨᒡᐦ ᐊᓂᔮᐦ ᐅᑎᓯᓃᒻᐦ, ᒫᓂᓈᔨᒡᐦ᙮

ᑏᐧᐋᐦᒡ ᓂᓯᑎᐧᐃᓈᑯᓂᔨᐤ ᐋᐦ ᒫᔮᑎᓂᔨᒡ ᐊᓂᔮ ᐅᔅᑳᑦ ᒑᒃ᙮ ᐋᐦ ᒥᓂᐱᔨᔨᒡᐦ ᐅᔑᑮᐦ ᑭᔮᐦ ᐋᐦ ᐹᑭᓂᔨᒡ, ᐋᐦ ᔓᔑᐧᐋᔨᒡ ᑭᔮᐦ ᐋᐦ ᒥᐦᐧᑳᔨᒡ ᑭᔮᐦ ᐋᐦ ᐱᒋᔅᑭᓈᔨᒡ᙮ ᐊᓂᑖᐦ ᐅᔮᐦᒡ ᐋᐦ ᐄᔅᐱᔨᔨᒡ ᐊᓂᔮᐦ ᐋᐦ ᒫᔮᑎᓂᔨᒡ ᐋᔪᐧᐃᒄ ᐧᐋᐦᒋ ᒌᐦ ᐧᐄᐦ ᐹᑯᒧᐧᐃᒥᒋᐦᐅᑦ ᒑᒃ᙮ ᑖᐹ ᐅᐦᒋ ᒋᔅᒑᔨᐦᑎᒻ ᒑᒃ ᐊᓂᔮ ᐋᐦ ᔖᑲᐅᐱᔨᑦ ᐋᔪᐧᐃᒄ ᐊᓂᔮ ᑳ ᐃᐦᑐᑖᑯᑦ ᐧᐋᐦᒋ ᐋᑳ ᐅᐦᒋ ᒌᐦ ᒦᓂᐧᐋᑎᓂᔨᒡ ᐊᓂᔮ ᐅᔅᑳᑦ; ᐋᑳ ᐅᐦᒋ ᒌᐦ ᐄᔥᐱᔒᒥᑭᓂᔨᒡ ᐊᓂᔮ ᐅᐲᔥᐲᔥᒃ ᒑ ᒌᐦ ᐅᔥᑖᒑᐱᔨᔨᒡ ᐊᓂᔮ ᒑᐧᑳᔨᐤ ᒑ ᒦᓂᐧᐋᒋᐦᐄᑯᑦ᙮ ᑳ ᒥᒥᔫᐦᑭᒥᔨᒡᐦ ᐊᓂᔮᐦ ᓂᑐᐦᑯᔨᓐᐦ ᐊᓂᔮ ᐅᔅᑳᑦ ᑭᔮᐦ ᑳ ᒥᔮᑭᓂᐧᐃᑦ ᒌᔥᑎᐦᐅᓂᑐᐦᑯᔨᓐᐦ᙮

ᒦᓐ ᒑᔅᒋᓯᑦ ᒑᒃ ᔖᔥ ᒥᒄ ᐊᓂᑖᐦ ᐧᒫᓐᑎᓅᐧᔮᑦ ᓂᑐᐦᑯᔨᓂᑭᒥᑯᐦᒡ ᐃᐦᑖᐤ᙮ ᐋᑯᑖᐦ ᑳ ᐄᑎᐦᐅᔮᑭᓂᐅᑯᐱᓈ ᐋᑳ ᓈᔥᑎᔨᒡ ᒋᔅᒋᓯᑦ᙮ ᓈᔥᒡ ᐋᐦᐧᑳᒡ ᐋᐦ ᒌᐦ ᐃᐦᑐᑖᑯᑦ ᐊᓂᔮ ᑳ

ᐹᑯᒧᐦᒋᐦᐅᑦ ᑲᔦ ᐁᑳ ᒣᒌ ᐃᑕᒪᐦᒋᐦᐅᑦ ᒧᐧᐁᐦᒡ ᐁᑳ ᓵᐸᒪᐦᒋᐦᐅᑦ ᒥᒄ ᑮᐹ ᒣᐧᑳᒡ ᐁ ᐊᔮᔅᐱᓰᐦᑳᓯᒪᑲᓂᔨᒡ ᐊᓂᔫ ᐅᔅᑳᑦ ᐁ ᒦᓂᐧᐋᒋᐦᐆᒪᑲᓂᔨᒡ ᒣᒌ ᐃᔥᐱᔥ ᒦᔮᑲᓅᑦ ᓂᑐᐦᑯᐃᓂᔫ᙮ ᑳ ᑲᓇᐧᐋᐸᒥᑯᑦ ᓂᑐᐦᑯᐃᓐ᙮ ᑳ ᐃᑎᑯᑦ, “ᓵᔅ ᓇᒧᐃ ᒋᐹ ᐅᐦᒋ ᒨᔑᐦᑖᓐ ᐊᓐ ᒋᔅᑳᑦ, ᑲᔦ ᒫᒃ ᓇᒧᐃ ᒋᐹ ᐅᐦᒋ ᒌᔅᐧᑫᔮᐱᒧᓐ ᑲᔦ ᓇᒧᐃ ᒋᐹ ᐅᐦᒋ ᐃᑕᒪᐦᒋᐦᐆᓐ ᒧᐧᐁᒡ ᐁᑳ ᓵᐸᒪᐦᒋᐦᐅᔨᓐ, ᓇᒧᐃ ᐃᐦᑑ ᐊᐧᐁᓐ ᒥᒄ ᐅᔅᑲᓐ ᐁᒌ ᓈᐧᑖᐦᑕᑖᑦ᙮ ᑳ ᐅᑎᓇᐦᒃ ᐊᓂᔫ ᒋᒧᐱᒑᑲᓂᔥ ᑳ ᐃᔑᓈᑯᓂᔨᒡ, ᑳ ᒪᓂᔕᒧᐧᐋᑦ ᐊᓂᔫ ᑳ ᐊᓯᓃᐦᑳᓂᐦᑲᐦᑌᔨᒡ, ᐁᒄ ᑳ ᐋᐸᐦᐄᐱᑕᐦᒃ᙮

ᒣᐧᑳᓐ ᐆ ᑳ ᒥᔫᓂᔨᒡ ᐊᓂᔫ ᒑᒃ ᐅᔅᑳᑦ᙮ ᓵᔅ ᒌ ᐹᐱᑯᒉᐸᔨᓂᔫ ᐁᒄ ᐧᐋᔅᑳ ᐊᓂᑕ ᑳ ᓈᐧᑖᐦᑎᓂᔨᒡ ᒌ ᐹᒋᐸᔨᓂᔫ ᒥᒍᓐ ᐁ ᔔᔓᐧᐋᔨᒡ ᑲᔦ ᒌ ᒥᐦᑯᐸᔨᓂᔫ, ᓵᔅ ᒌᐧᐄ ᐧᐄᐱᐸᔨᓂᔫ ᐊᓂᔫ ᐅᔅᑳᑦ᙮ ᐁᐅᒄ ᒫᒃ ᐊᓂᔫ ᑳ ᐃᐦᑑᑖᑯᑦ ᒑᒃ ᐧᐁᐦᒌ ᒌᔥᐧᑫᔮᐸᒧᑦ ᒨᔥ᙮ ᓇᒧᐃ ᑮᐹ ᐅᐦᒋ ᒋᔅᒣᔨᐦᑕᒻ, ᐊᓂᔫ ᐁ ᓰᐧᐋᑲᒥᐦᐧᑫᑦ ᐁᐅᒄ ᐊᓂᔫ ᐧᐁᐦᒋ ᐁᑳ ᐅᐦᒌ ᒥᐧᔮᔨᒡ ᐊᓂᔫ ᐅᔅᑳᑦ᙮ ᐊᓂᔫ ᐅᐦᐹᐱᑯᓰᒻ ᐧᐁᓵ ᓰᒃ ᐁᒌ ᐋᐸᑎᓰᒪᑲᓂᔨᒡ ᐁ ᐧᐄ ᐅᔑᑖᒣᒪᑲᓂᔨᒡ ᐊᓂᔫ ᒣᐧᑳᔫ ᓀᑐᐧᐁᔨᐦᑖᑯᓂᔨᒡ ᒣᒌ ᐅᐦᒋ ᒦᓄᐧᐋᑎᓰᑦ᙮ ᑳ ᐸᔦᐦᒋᐦᐧᐋᔨᒡ ᓂᑐᐦᑯᐃᓐ ᐊᓂᔫ ᐅᔅᑲᐃ ᐁᒄ ᑳ ᒦᑯᑦ ᐁ ᓂᑐᐦᑯᐃᓈᐴᓂᔨᐧᑳᐤ ᓂᑐᐦᑯᐃᓐ ᒣᒌ ᐄᒣᐸᔨᓂᔨᒡ ᐊᓂᔫ ᑳ ᒥᔫᓂᔨᒡ᙮

ᒣᒃ ᐯᔭᐧᑳᐤ ᒌ ᒥᔅᑳᑎᓰ ᒑᒃ ᐧᐋᐦᔫ ᐊᓂᑌ ᒥᐦᒣᑐ ᐊᔅᒌᐤ ᑎᐸᐦᐄᑲᓐᐦ ᐁ ᐃᐦᑖᑦ, ᒨᓕᔮᐦᒡ ᐁ ᒌ ᐃᑎᔑᐦᐧᐋᑲᓅᑯᐸᓄ᙮ ᑳᐱᒥᐦᔮᒪᑲᓂᔨᒡ ᐁᒌ ᐋᐸᑕᓂᔨᑯᐸᓄ᙮ ᓇᒧᐃ ᒫᒃ ᒥᒍᓐ ᐅᐦᒋ ᒋᔅᒋᓰ

une pilule pour contrôler ses nausées et sa faiblesse pendant que sa jambe guérissait. Le médecin le regarda curieusement. Selon le médecin, la douleur aurait dû s'atténuer depuis longtemps et, de plus, les nausées et la faiblesse *n'étaient* pas des symptômes de fractures. Il attrapa sa petite scie électrique, scia le plâtre et l'enleva.

subsided long ago, the doctor said, and nausea and weakness were *not* actually symptoms of broken bones. He reached for his small electric saw, sawed off the cast, and lifted it away.

La jambe de Jack était manifestement infectée. La peau pelait et la zone autour de la fracture était enflée, brillante, rouge, violette et verte. L'infection avait saturé le corps Jack de toxines, ce qui lui donnait la nausée. Jack ne le savait pas, mais son diabète l'empêchait de guérir; son pancréas était trop épuisé pour créer les hormones qui aident le corps à guérir. Le médecin nettoya la peau et donna des antibiotiques à Jack pour combattre l'infection...

Jack's leg was obviously infected. The skin was peeling and the area around the break was swollen and shiny and red and purple and green. The infection had filled Jack with toxins and was making him nauseous. Jack didn't know it, but his diabetes was preventing healing; his pancreas was too burned out to create the hormones that help the body heal. The doctor cleaned up the skin, gave Jack antibiotics for the infection...

... Et Jack se réveilla à des centaines de kilomètres de là, à l'hôpital de Montréal. Il y avait été transporté par avion. Il ne se souvenait de rien. L'infection de sa

...And Jack woke up hundreds of kilometres away in the hospital in Montréal. He had been airlifted there. He remembered none of it. The infection in

ᒫᔮᑎᓂᔨᒡ ᐅᔅᑳᑦ ᐊᓂᑖᐦ ᐅᒥᐦᑯᐦᒡ ᐋᐦ ᒌᐦ ᐄᔅᐱᔨᔨᒡ ᑮᔮᐦ ᓂᒥ ᐧᐋᐧᐋᒡ ᔖᔥ ᑯᐃᔅᒄ ᐅᐦᒋ ᒌᐦ ᐄᔑ ᒫᒥᑐᓈᔨᐦᑎᒻ᙮

ᐄᔅᑯᑎᒃ ᑳ ᑯᔥᑯᐱᔨᑦ ᒑᒃ ᑮᔮᐦ ᒋᔥᒋᐧᐋ ᑳ ᐧᐋᔅᑭᒫᔨᑎᐦᒃ, ᑳ ᐧᐄᐦᑎᒫᑯᑦ ᐊᓂᔮᐦ ᓂᑐᐦᑯᑯᔨᓐᐦ ᐊᓂᔮᐦ ᑳ ᑎᐦᑯᐦᐅᑯᑦ ᐊᓂᔮᐦ ᐅᒑᐸᓈᔥᑯᔥᐦ, ᐋᑳ ᑯᐃᔅᒄ ᐅᐦᒋ ᑖᐱᒧᐦᑖᔨᒡᐦ ᐊᓂᔮ ᐅᔅᑳᑦ ᐊᓂᔮᐦ ᓂᑐᐦᑯᔨᓐᐦ ᑳ ᒋᑭᒧᐦᐋᔨᒡᐦ ᐊᓂᔮᐦ ᐅᑎᓯᓃᒻᐦ ᐊᓂᑎᐦ ᐅᔅᑳᑎᐦᒡ᙮ ᔖᔥ ᒫᒃ ᒥᐦᒑᑐ ᐲᓯᒻ ᓂᒥ ᐅᐦᒋ ᒥᐧᔮᔨᐤ ᐊᓂᔮ ᐅᔅᑳᑦ ᐋᑳ ᑯᐃᔅᒄ ᐅᐦᒋ ᑖᐱᒧᐦᑖᑭᓂᐧᐃᐧᐃᔨᒡ ᐊᓂᑎᐦ ᑳ ᓈᐧᑖᐱᔨᔨᒡ ᐊᓂᔮ ᐅᔅᑳᑦ ᑮᔮᐦ ᐊᓂᔮ ᐋᐦ ᔖᑲᐅᐱᔨᑦ, ᓈᔥᑎᔨᒡ ᐋᑳ ᐅᐦᒋ ᐊᑎ ᒥᐧᔮᔨᒡ ᑮᔮᐦ ᐋᔥᒄ ᐋᐦ ᒌᐦ ᓈᐧᑖᐱᔨᔨᒡ ᑮᔮᐦ ᐋᔥᒄ ᐋᐦ ᒌᐦ ᒫᔮᑎᓂᔨᒡ᙮ ᒦᓐ ᑳ ᑖᐱᒧᐦᑖᑭᓂᐧᐃᐧᐃᔨᒡ ᐊᓂᔮ ᐅᔅᑭᓐ ᑮᔮᐦ ᒦᓐ ᑳ ᐧᐄᐦ ᒦᓂᐧᐋᒋᐦᑖᑭᓂᐧᐃᐧᐃᔨᒡ᙮ ᐊᓂᑖᐦ ᒫᒃ ᐋᐦ ᐅᔮᓯᐧᐃᔨᒡ ᐊᓂᔮ ᐅᔅᑳᑦ ᐋᑯᑖᐦ ᑳ ᐄᔑ ᒋᑭᒧᐦᑖᑭᓂᐧᐃᐧᐃᔨᒡ ᒑᐧᑳᔨᐤ ᐊᓂᑎᐦ ᒑ ᒌ ᐅᐦᒋ ᑯᐃᐧᑳᔑᑭᐧᐃᐧᐃᔨᒡ ᐊᓂᔮ ᐋᐦ ᒦᐅᐧᐃᔨᒡ ᑮᔮᐦ ᒑ ᐧᐃᔨᐧᐄᔮᐳᑖᔨᒡ ᐊᓂᔮ ᒑᐧᑳᔨᐤ ᐋᐦ ᒫᔮᑎᓂᔨᒡ ᐊᓂᑖᐦ ᐲᐦᒡ ᑳ ᐃᐦᑎᑯᓂᔨᒡ᙮ ᐋᓯᐦᒡ ᒌᐦ ᐋᐦᑎᒧᐦᑖᑭᓂᐧᐃᐧᐃᔨᐤᐦ ᐊᓂᔮᐦ ᐅᒥᒌᐧᐋᒋᓐᐦ ᑮᔮᐦ ᓈᔥᒡ ᑯᐃᔅᒄ ᒨᔥ ᒌᐦ ᐧᐄᐦ ᐱᔮᐦᒋᐦᐋᑭᓂᐧᐃᐧᐃᔨᐤᐦ ᐊᓂᔮᐦ ᐅᔑᑮᐦ᙮

ᓈᔥᒡ ᐋᐦ ᒌᐦ ᒥᒑᔨᐦᑎᐦᒃ ᒑᒃ ᒥᒄ ᐋᐦ ᐋᔨᐱᑦ᙮ ᐊᓂᑎᐦ ᒫᒃ ᐊᓂᔮ ᐧᒫᓐᑎᓅᐧᔮᑦ ᓂᑐᐦᑯᔨᓂᑭᒥᑯᔨᐤ ᒌᐦ ᒥᐦᒑᑎᔨᐤᐦ ᑯᑎᒃᐦ ᐄᔨᔨᐤᐦ, ᑳ ᒌᐦ ᐱᐹᒥᐱᔨᑦ ᐋᐦ ᓂᑑᒨᒋᔕᒪᑦ ᙮ ᐱᔥᒡ ᐊᓂᔮᐦ ᑖᐹ ᐅᐦᒋ ᑭᔅᒋᐦᐅᔨᐤᐦ

ᐅᔫ ᑳ ᐃᐦᑑᑐᐧᐋᑲᓅᑯᐸᓀ᙮ ᐊᓂᔫ ᐅᔅᑳᑦ ᐁ ᒥᔫᓂᔨᒡ ᒥᔅᑕᐦᐄ ᐅᒥᐦᑯᐦᒡ ᒌ ᐃᔅᐸᔨᓂᔫ ᒥᒍᓐ ᐁᒌ ᐧᐄᓈᑲᒥᐸᔨᔨᒡ ᐅᒥᐦᒄ ᐁᐅᒄ ᑮᐹ ᐅᔫ ᑳ ᐃᐦᑑᑖᑯᑦ ᐧᐁᐦᒌ ᐁᑳ ᐱᔦᑭᔅᒋᒫᒥᑐᓀᔨᐦᑕᐦᒃ᙮

ᐃᔅᑯᑕᒃ ᒫᒃ ᑳ ᐋᐱᔅᑯᔑᑦ ᐁ ᐊᑎ ᐧᐋᔅᑲᒣᔨᒨᑦ ᒫᒃ, ᒌ ᐃᑎᑰ ᐊᓂᔫ ᓂᑐᐦᑯᐃᓐ ᐊᓂᑕ ᒧᓚᔮᐦᒡ ᑳ ᐃᐦᑖᔨᒡ ᐁᑳ ᒧᔮᒻ ᐅᐦᒋ ᐃᐦᑑᑕᒥᔨᑯᐸᓀᓐ ᐊᓂᔫᐦ ᓂᑐᐦᑯᐄᓐ ᑳ ᐱᒦᐦᑲᒥᔨᒡ ᐊᓂᔫ ᐅᔅᑳᑦ ᓀᑌ ᐁᐃᒧᔅ ᑳ ᐃᐦᑖᔨᒡ᙮ ᒥᒉᑐ ᐲᓯᒻ ᒌᐧᐄ ᒦᓂᐧᐋᒋᐦᐆᒪᑲᓂᔫ ᐊᓂᔫ ᐅᔅᑳᑦ ᓇᒧᐃ ᐅᐦᒋ ᐃᐦᐄᓂᔫ ᐊᓂᔫ ᐅᐦᒋ ᐁᑳ ᒧᔮᒻ ᐅᐦᒋ ᐃᐦᑑᑖᑲᓅᔨᒡ ᑲᔦ ᒫᒃ ᐁ ᓰᐧᐋᑲᒥᐦᐧᑫᑦ᙮ ᓇᒧᐃ ᒥᒍᓐ ᐅᐦᒌ ᒥᐧᔮᔫ ᑲᔦ ᐁᔅᒄ ᐁᑯᓐ ᑳ ᐃᔑᓈᑯᓂᔨᒡ ᐊᓂᔫ ᐅᔅᑳᑎᑲᓐ ᐁᑳ ᒥᒍᓐ ᐅᐦᒋ ᐊᑎ ᒥᐧᔮᔨᑯᐸᓀ ᑲᔦ ᐁᔅᒄ ᒥᔅᑕᐦᐄ ᒌ ᒥᔫᓂᔫ᙮ ᐁᒄ ᒦᓐ ᑳ ᑖᐱᐦᑕᑖᑲᓅᔨᒡ ᐊᓂᑕ ᑳ ᓈᐧᑖᐸᔨᓂᔨᒡ ᐁᐧᐄ ᐧᐄᒋᐦᑖᑲᓅᔨᒡ ᑫᒌ ᒥᐧᔮᔨᒡ᙮ ᐅᑎᒋᔑᔮᐱᒻ ᐁ ᔖᑯᐧᐋᐯᑲᔑᐧᑳᐤ ᒌ ᐱᐦᑕᐱᐦᑫᓂᑲᓅᔫᐦ ᓂᑖᒥᐦᒡ ᐅᔅᑳᐦᒡ ᐁᒄ ᑳ ᐅᑕᐦᐄᑲᓅᔨᒡ ᐊᓂᔫ ᒥᔨᔨᔫ ᐁᑳ ᐁᑎᑑ ᑫᒌ ᐅᔑᐦᐆᒪᑲᓂᔨᒡ ᐊᓂᑕ ᐅᔅᑳᑎᐦᒡ᙮ ᒨᔥ ᒌ ᐋᐦᑕᒧᐦᑖᑲᓅᔫ ᐊᓂᔫ ᐅᒫᐦᑯᐱᒋᑲᓐ ᑲᔦ ᐧᐁᐧᐁᐃᑦ ᒌ ᑲᓇᐧᐋᐸᐦᑖᑲᓅᔫ ᒫᓐᐦ ᐊᓂᑕᐦ ᑳ ᒥᔫᓂᔨᒡ ᐊᓂᔫ ᐅᔅᑳᑦ᙮

ᓈᔅᒡ ᐁᒌ ᒪᑫᔨᐦᑕᐦᒃ ᐁᑳ ᐧᐃᔦᔅ ᒌ ᐃᐦᑎᑦ ᒥᒄ ᐁ ᐊᔭᐱᑦ᙮ ᐊᓂᑕ ᒧᓚᔮᐦᒡ ᐋᐦᑯᓰᐅᑲᒥᑯᐦᒡ ᑳ ᐃᐦᑖᑦ ᒌ ᒥᐦᑫᑎᔦ ᑯᑕᒃ ᐄᓅ ᐋᐦᑯᓯᐅᐄᓅᐦ ᐊᓂᑕ ᐁ ᐃᐦᑖᔨᐧᑖᐤ ᐁᐊᒄ ᑳᒌ ᐸᐹᑯᐦᑯᐦᐆᓯᑦ ᐁ ᑲᒋᔦᑕᒫᑦ᙮ ᐸᔅᒡ ᓇᒧᐃ ᐅᐦᒋ ᑲᔅᒋᐦᐅᔦᐦ ᐁ

jambe cassée avait tellement empoisonné son sang qu'elle avait même affecté sa capacité à penser.

his broken leg had poisoned his blood so badly that it had even affected his ability to think.

Une fois Jack complètement réveillé et alerte, le médecin de Montréal lui dit que, le jour de l'accident, le médecin d'Amos n'avait pas réduit correctement la fracture de sa jambe. L'os essayait de guérir depuis des mois désormais, mais, à cause de la mauvaise réduction de la fracture et de son diabète, la guérison n'avait pas du tout progressé et l'os était toujours aussi cassé et infecté. Ils repositionnèrent l'os et tentèrent de donner à sa jambe une nouvelle chance de guérir. Ils insérèrent – directement dans la chair – des tubes étroits pour aspirer le pus et les fluides supplémentaires en dehors de la jambe pour que ceux-là ne puissent pas emprisonner de toxines dans le corps. Ils changèrent souvent ses pansements, en vérifiant toujours très attentivement la chair en voie de guérison.

Once Jack was fully awake and alert again, the Montréal doctor told him that, way back on the day of the accident, the doctor in Amos hadn't set the broken leg properly. The bone had been trying to heal for months now, but, because of the improper bone setting and because of his diabetes, it had made no headway at all and was as broken and infected as ever. They re-set the bone then and tried to give the leg another chance to heal. They inserted – right into the flesh – narrow tubes that collected the extra pus and fluids and carried them out of the leg so they couldn't trap toxins inside. They changed the bandages often, always checking the healing flesh very carefully.

Jack détestait rester assis sans bouger. Dans cet hôpital de Montréal, il y avait beaucoup d'autres Cris, alors il passait le temps en se déplaçant en fauteuil roulant pour leur rendre visite. Certains

Jack hated sitting still. In this Montréal hospital were many other Cree people, so he passed the time by wheeling himself around and visiting them. Some of the older ones didn't speak English or French

ᐋᐦ ᐧᐋᒥᔥᑎᑯᔒᐅᔨᒥᔨᒡᐦ ᑭᔮᐦ ᒫᒃ ᐋᐦ ᐱᔥᑎᐧᑳᔮᐅᔨᒥᔨᒡᐦ ᑭᔮᐦ ᓈᔥᒡ ᐋᐦ ᒌᐦ ᒥᔮᔨᐦᑎᐦᒡᐦ ᐋᐦ ᐹᐦᑎᐧᐋᒡ ᐊᐧᐋᔨᐤᐦ ᐋᐦ ᐄᔨᔨᐅᔨᒥᔨᒡᐦ᙮ ᑏᐧᐋᐦᒡ ᒫᒃ ᑳᐦ ᒋᔅᒑᔨᒥᑯᑦ ᒑᒃ ᑏᐧᐋᐦᒡ ᒌᐦ ᐋᐱᒋᐦᐄᑰ ᒑ ᐄᐧᑖᔥᑎᒧᐧᐋᑦ ᐊᓂᔮᐦ ᐅᑖᐦᑯᓯᐤᐦ ᐋᑳ ᒌᐦ ᐊᔨᒦᔥᑎᒫᓯᔨᒡᐦ᙮ ᒨᔥ ᒫᒃ ᑳ ᐃᐦᑎᒃ ᒑᒃ ᐋᐦ ᓂᑎᐧᐋᐱᒫᑦ ᐊᓂᔮᐦ ᑯᑎᒃᐦ ᐄᔨᔨᐤᐦ ᐋᐦ ᒨᒋᔖᒫᑦ ᑭᔮᐦ ᐋᐦ ᐄᔨᔨᐅᔨᒥᐦᐋᑦ ᐋᑳ ᓈᔥᒡ ᒑ ᒌᐦ ᒋᔅᒋᓰᑎᑎᒥᔨᒡᐦ ᐊᓂᔮᐦ ᐋᐦ ᒫᓂᑖᐧᐋᔨᐦᑎᒥᔨᒡᐦ ᐋᑎ ᐃᔨᐦᑐᑎᐧᐋᑭᓂᐧᐃᐧᐃᔨᒡᐦ ᑭᔮᐦ ᐋᑳ ᓈᔥᒡ ᒑ ᔅᒑᔨᐦᑎᒥᔨᒡᐦ᙮ (ᑖᓂᑖᐦ ᒫᒃ ᑳ ᐃᐦᑎᒡ ᐊᓂᒌ ᒋᔖᔨᔨᐅᒡ ᒫᐧᑳᒡ ᐋᑳ ᐃᐦᑖᔨᒡᐦ ᐊᐧᐋᔨᐤᐦ ᒑ ᐄᐧᑖᔥᑎᒫᑯᒡ, ᑳᑭᔮᐦ ᒥᒄ ᓂᒥ ᐅᐦᒋ ᒌᐦ ᒋᔅᑐᐧᐃᒡ ᒑ ᒌᐦ ᐧᐄᐦᑎᐦᒡᐦ ᐋᑳ ᒫᔪᐱᔨᐦᐄᑯᐧᑖᐤᐦ ᒑᐧᑳᔨᐤ᙮)

ᐧᐁᒥᔅᑎᑰᓰᐅᐊᔨᒥᔨᒡ ᒫᒃ ᐁ ᑳᑯᔅᑫᓯᐅᐊᔨᒥᔨᒡ ᐁᒄ ᓈᔅᒡ ᑳ ᒥᔦᔨᐦᑕᐦᐧᑳᐤ ᐁ ᐃᐦᑖᔨᒡ ᐊᐧᐁᔫ ᐁ ᐄᓅᐊᔨᒥᔨᒡ᙮ ᑫᒃ ᒌ ᐧᐋᐸᐦᑕᒥᔫ ᓂᑐᐦᑯᐃᓂᔅᐧᑫᐤᐦ ᑲᔦ ᓂᑐᐦᑯᐃᓐ ᑖᓐ ᐁ ᐃᔑ ᑲᔅᒋᐦᐅᑦ ᒑᒃ ᐁᒄ ᑳᒌ ᐧᐄᔖᒪᐧᑖᐤ ᒫᓐᐦ ᑫᒌ ᐧᐄᐦᑕᒧᐧᐋᔨᒡ ᐊᐧᐁᔫᐦ ᒥᒄ ᑳ ᐄᓅᐊᔨᒥᔨᒡ ᑖᓐ ᑫ ᐃᔑ ᓂᑐᐦᑯᐦᐋᑲᓅᔨᒡ᙮ ᑳᒌ ᑯᐦᑯᐦᐅᓯᑦ ᐊᓂᑌ ᐃᔑ ᑫᒌ ᓂᑑ ᐃᐧᑌᔥᑕᒧᐧᐋᑦ ᐊᓂᔫ ᐋᐦᑯᓰᐅᐄᓅᐦ ᓂᑐᐦᑯᐃᓐᐦ ᐁᐧᐄ ᐊᔨᒥᐦᐄᑯᔨᒡ᙮ ᐁᑯᓐ ᑳᒌ ᐃᐦᑎᑦ ᐁ ᓇᓂᑐᐧᐋᐸᒫᑦ ᐊᓂᔫᐦ ᐋᐦᑯᓰᐅᐄᓅᐦ ᐁᒄ ᑳᒌ ᐹᐦᐱᐦᐋᑦ ᐁ ᑎᐹᒋᒧᔥᑕᐧᐋᑦ ᐁᒄ ᓇᒧᐃ ᐅᐦᒋ ᐃᔥᐱᔥ ᐋᐃᒉᔨᐦᑕᒥᔫᐦ ᑖᓐ ᑫ ᐃᐦᑑᑖᑯᔨᒡ ᓂᑐᐦᑯᐄᓐᐦ ᑲᔦ ᓇᒧᐃ ᐅᐦᒋ ᐃᔥᐱᔥ ᔅᒋᓰᒡ ᐊᓂᑕ ᐁ ᐃᐦᑖᐧᑖᐤ᙮ ᓈᔅᒡ ᑖᐧᐯ ᒌ ᒥᔦᔨᐦᑕᒻ ᒑᒃ ᐅᔫ ᐁ ᐃᔑ ᐧᐄᒋᐦᐋᑦ ᐊᓂᔫᐦ ᐋᐦᑯᓰᐅᐄᓅᐦ᙮ (ᐁᐃᔑ ᒫ ᐃᐦᑑᒡ ᒋᒐᐃᓅᒡ ᐁᑳ ᐃᐦᑖᔨᒡ ᐊᐧᐁᔫ ᑫᒌ ᐃᐧᑌᔥᑕᒫᑯᐧᑖᐤ᙮ ᔅᒋᓰᑫᓂᒡ ᑮᐹ ᓈᓂᑑ ᐁᑳ ᒌ ᐊᔨᒥᐦᐋᐧᑖᐤ ᐊᐧᐁᔫᐦ)᙮

ᒑᒃ ᑭᔨᐧᐹ ᐹᑎᒫᐦ ᒦᓐ ᑳ ᒌᐧᐋᑦ ᒑᒃ ᓈᑖᐦ ᐄᔑ ᐧᐋᐧᓵᓂᐲᐦᒡ, ᑭᔮᐦ ᒨᔥ ᑳ ᐄᑐᐦᑖᑦ ᐊᓂᑖᐦ ᓂᑐᐦᑯᔨᓂᑭᒥᑯᐦᒡ ᒑ ᓈᓈᑭᒋᐦᐋᑭᓂᐧᐃᑦ ᑭᔮᐦ ᒑ ᓂᑑᑏᐹᔨᒫᑭᓂᐧᐃᑦ᙮ ᐹᔨᐧᑳᐤ ᐋᐦ ᒌᔑᑳᔨᒡ ᒫᐧᑳᒡ ᐋᐦ ᐱᐹᒫᔅᑭᐦᐅᓯᑦ ᐊᓂᑖᐦ ᓂᑐᐦᑯᔨᓂᑭᒥᑯᐦᒡ, ᑳᐦ ᔖᔥᑯᐱᔨᑦ ᐊᓂᑎᐦ ᓈᐦᐋᐤ ᐋᐦ ᓂᐲᐧᐃᔨᒡ ᓂᐱᒋᔅᑎᑯᔨᐤ ᑭᔮᐦ ᑳᐦ ᐱᐦᒋᔑᐦᒃ᙮

ᑫᒃ ᒫᒃ ᒌ ᒌᐧᐁᐤ ᑳᐤ ᐧᐋᔅᐧᐋᓂᐲᐦᒡ ᑳᒌ ᐃᑐᐦᑌᑦ ᒫᓐᐦ ᓂᑐᐦᑯᐃᓂᑲᒥᑯᐦᒡ ᑫᒌ ᑲᓇᐧᐋᐸᐦᑖᑲᓅᔨᒡ ᐊᓂᔫ ᐅᔅᑳᑦ᙮ ᐯᔭᐧᑳᐤ ᒫᒃ, ᐁ ᐄᑑ ᓴᔅᑲᐦᐅᑦ ᒌ ᑖᐅᐦᐊᒻ ᐁ ᓂᐲᐅᐦᑕᑳᔨᒡ ᐁᒄ ᑳ ᓰᔅᑯᐸᔨᑦ ᑳ ᐋᐧᑫᔨᐦᑕᐦᒃ᙮

des plus âgés ne parlaient ni anglais ni français et étaient très reconnaissants d'avoir quelqu'un avec qui parler dans leur propre langue. Il ne fallut que peu de temps pour que les médecins et les infirmières se rendent compte de ce que Jack pouvait faire et, bientôt, ils vinrent le chercher chaque fois qu'ils devaient avoir une intervention sur un Cri qui ne parlait pas leur langue. Jack se déplaçait en fauteuil roulant dans la pièce et traduisait pour les médecins et les patients cris. Pendant tout ce temps, il rendait aussi visite aux Cris et plaisantait avec eux dans leur propre langue pour leur faire oublier toutes ces procédures étranges et cet endroit effrayant dans lequel ils se trouvaient. C'était tellement bon de se sentir à nouveau utile. (Mais que faisaient tous les Cris âgés quand il n'y avait personne pour traduire pour eux ? Souffraient-ils simplement dans la peur et le silence ?)

Finalement, Jack rentra chez lui à Waswanipi, où il se rendit consciencieusement et régulièrement à la clinique pour des examens. Un jour, alors qu'il se déplaçait avec des béquilles dans les couloirs, il glissa sur un coin de sol mouillé.

and were so grateful to have someone there to talk with in their own language. It didn't take long at all for the doctors and nurses to realize what Jack could do, and soon they came for him whenever they had to do a procedure on a Cree person who couldn't speak their languages. Jack wheeled himself into the room and translated for the doctors and the Cree patients. All the while, he visited and joked with the Cree folks in their own language to take their minds off of all of these strange procedures and of the scary place they were in. It felt so good to be useful again. (But what did all the elderly Cree do when no one was there to translate for them? Did they just suffer in fear and silence?)

Eventually, Jack went back home to Waswanipi, where he dutifully stopped by the clinic regularly for check-ups. One day, making his way on crutches around the halls, he hit a patch of wet floor and wiped right out.

ᐧᐋᐦᒋ ᒥᐧᑖᑮᓈᐱᔨᔨᒡ ᒑᐧᑳᔨᐤ!

ᓈᔥᒡ ᐋᐦ ᒫᑯᐦᐄᑯᑦ ᐊᓂᔮ ᐅᔅᑳᑦ ᐋᑲ ᐅᐦᒋ ᐅᔮᔑᓂᔨᒡ ᑮᔮᐦ ᒑᔅᒋᓯᑦ ᒦᓐ ᐋᐦ ᒌᐦ ᐄᔑ ᒨᔑᐦᑖᑦ ᐅᔮ. ᑳ ᐋᐦᑯᐦᑎᑖᑦ ᐅᐦᒋᑯᓐ, ᐊᓂᔮᐦ ᐋᑲ ᐧᐋᐦᒋ ᐋᐦᑯᓯᑦ. ᐅᐧᐋ, ᓂᐧᐃᒡ ᓂᒥ ᐅᐦᒋ ᒥᔦᐱᔨᐦᐄᑰ ᒑᐧᑳᔨᐤ.

ᓈᑖᐦ ᑳ ᐄᒋᔑᐦᐅᑯᑦ ᓂᑐᐦᑯᔨᓐᐦ ᔑᐳᑯᒨ ᓂᑐᐦᑯᔨᓂᑭᒥᑯᐦᐦᒡ ᐋᑯᑎᐦ ᑳ ᒋᑭᒧᐦᑖᔨᒡᐦ ᒫᒋᔑᒑᓯᐤᐦ ᒑᐧᑳᔨᐤ ᐊᓂᑎᐦ ᐅᐦᒋᑯᓂᐦᐦᒡ ᒐ ᒌᐦ ᒌᑐᐱᔨᔨᒡ ᑮᔮᐦ ᒐ ᒌᐦ ᒦᓂᐧᐋᑎᓂᔨᒡ. ᓈᐅᔥ ᒫᒃ ᒌᐦ ᔔᔔᐧᐄᐤ ᑮᔮᐦ ᒌᐦ ᐧᐄᒋᐦᐋᑭᓂᐤ ᐋᐦ ᔮᔮᐦᒋᐱᑎᑭᓂᐧᐃᐧᐃᔨᒡ ᐊᓂᔮᐦ ᐅᐦᒋᑯᓐ, ᑮᔮᐦ ᒑᒃ ᐋᑎᐧᐄ ᑳ ᐋᑎ ᒦᓂᐧᐋᑎᓂᔨᒡ ᐊᓂᔮ ᐅᔅᑳᑦ.

ᐋᑯᐦ ᐊᓂᔮ ᑯᑎᒋᔨᐤ ᐅᔅᑳᑦ, ᐊᓂᔮ ᑳ ᓈᐧᑖᐱᔨᔨᒡ ᑳ ᑎᑭᐦᐅᑯᑦ ᐅᒑᐸᓈᔥᑯᔥᐦ, ᐋᔮᐱᒡ ᒨᔥ ᒌᐦ ᐋᐦᑯᓯᐤ. ᐹᔨᐧᑲᐤ ᐋᐦ ᐅᑖᑯᔑᔨᒡ, ᑳ ᒌᔑ ᒦᒋᓯᒡ, ᓈᔥᒡ ᒥᒄ ᓂᑎᐧᐄ ᐋᐦ ᐄᔑ ᐊᔨᒥᐦᐋᑦ ᐅᑳᐧᐄᐦ ᐋᑲ ᓈᔥᑎᔨᒡ ᓂᓯᑐᐦᑖᑯᑦ. ᓈᔥᒡ ᓰᐦᐦᒃ ᐋᐦ ᑭᓂᐧᐋᐱᒥᑯᑦ, ᐹᔓᒡ ᐅᑖᔥᑎᒥᐦᑯᐦᐦᒡ = ᑏᐧᐋᐦᐦᒡ ᒌᐦ ᒥᐧᑖᐦᑖᔨᐤᐦ ᒑ ᐹᒋ ᓈᑎᐦᐧᐋᑭᓂᐧᐃᑦ. ᑏᐧᐋᐦᐦᒡ ᐧᒫᓐᑎᓅᐧᔮᑦ ᒌᐦ ᐄᑎᔑᐦᐆᑯᑦ ᓂᑐᐦᑯᔨᓐᐦ ᑳ ᐱᐹᒥᐦᔮᒥᑭᓂᔨᒡ ᐋᐦ ᐋᐱᑎᓂᔨᒡ.

ᓈᔥᑎᔨᒡ ᓂᒥ ᐅᐦᒋ ᒌᐦ ᒥᐧᔮᔨᐤ ᐊᓂᔮ ᐅᔅᑲ ᒑᒃ. ᔔᔥ ᑯᐧᑖᔥᒡ ᑎᐦᑐ ᐲᓯᒼ, ᐋᑦ ᐧᐄᐦ

ᒨᔑᐦᑖᑦ ᐧᐃᔦᔅ ᐁ ᐃᔅᐸᔨᑦ.

ᐊᓂᔫ ᑳ ᒥᐧᔮᔨᒡ ᐅᔅᑳᑦ ᐧᐃᔦᔅ ᒌ ᐃᔑᐦᑕᑖᐤ. ᓇᐦᐋᐤ ᐅᐦᒋᑯᓂᐦᐦᒡ ᐁᑯᑦ ᑳ ᒨᔑᐦᑖᑦ ᐧᐃᔦᔅ ᐁ ᐃᔅᐸᔨᓂᔨᒡ. ᒌ ᐲᑯᐦᑎᓂᔨᑯᐸᓄ ᒫᒃ. ᑖᐧᐯᐦ ᓇᒧᐃ ᓂᒋᐦᑳᐧᐋᒋᐸᔨᓐ ᒌ ᐃᑌᔨᐦᑕᒼ.

ᔑᐳᑲᒨ ᐋᐦᑯᓰᐅᑲᒥᑯᐦᐦᒡ ᒌ ᐄᑎᔑᐦᐆᑰ ᓂᑐᐦᑯᐃᓐ ᐋᐦᑯᓰᐅᑖᐹᓂᔫ ᐁᒌ ᐋᐸᒋᐦᑖᑦ ᐁᑯᑌ ᑳ ᐧᐁᔥᑖᑲᓅᔨᒡ ᐊᓂᔫ ᐅᐦᒋᑯᓐ, ᐱᐧᔮᐱᔅᑯᔫ ᐁᒌ ᒋᑲᒧᐦᑖᑲᓅᔨᒡ ᐁᑳ ᒉᒌ ᐋᐦᒋᐸᔨᓂᔨᒡ ᐊᓂᑕ ᓇᐦᐋᐤ ᐊᓂᔫ ᐅᐦᒋᑯᓐ ᐧᐄᐸᒡ ᒉᒌ ᒥᐧᔮᔨᒡ. ᐃᔅᑯᑖᒃ ᒫᒃ ᒉᐧᔮᔨᒡ ᐁᒄ ᑲᒌ ᓂᑑ ᓴᓵᐅᐸᔨᐦᑖᑦ ᐊᓂᔫ ᐅᔅᑳᑦ ᒦᓐ ᑳᐤ ᒉᒌ ᐱᒧᐦᑌᐧᐋᒉᑦ. ᒥᐦᒉᑐ ᑑᔥᑌᐤᐦ ᐁᑯᓐ ᒨᔥ ᑳ ᐃᐦᑎᑦ ᐁ ᐃᑐᐦᑌᑦ ᐊᓂᑌ ᐁ ᐅᐦᒋ ᐧᐄᒋᐦᐋᑲᓅᑦ, ᒉᒃ ᒫᒃ ᑌᑭᔥ ᒌ ᒥᐧᔮᔫ ᐊᓂᔫ ᐅᐦᒋᑯᓐ.

ᐊᓂᔫ ᐧᐄ ᑯᑕᒋᔫ ᐅᔅᑳᑦ ᑳ ᓈᐧᑖᐦᑕᑖᑦ ᑳ ᑯᑕᐸᔨᓂᔑᐧᐋᐤ ᐅᑖᐹᓂᔑᐧᐋᐤ ᐁᔅᒄ ᔮᐸᒡ ᒌ ᐋᐦᑯᓰ. ᐯᔭᐧᑳᐤ ᒫᒃ ᐁ ᐅᑖᑯᔑᔨᒡ ᑳ ᐃᔅᐧᑳᐤ ᒦᒋᓯᐧᑖᐤ, ᒉᐧᑳᒡ ᐁ ᐊᔨᒥᐦᐋᑦ ᐅᑳᐧᐃ ᒉᒃ ᓇᒧᐃ ᐅᐦᒋ ᑲᒋᐦᑳᐧᐋᔅᑖᑯᓰ ᑖᓐ ᐁ ᐃᐧᑌᑦ. ᑳ ᐧᐋᐸᐦᑕᒥᔨᒡ ᐅᔅᒌᔑᒄᐦ ᐁᑳ ᒨᔭᒼ ᐃᑕᑯᑎᓂᔨᐧᑳᐤ ᐁᒄ ᑳ ᑖᐦᑲᐱᐦᒉᓂᒉᑦ ᒉᒌ ᐹᐸᔨᓂᔨᒡ ᐋᐦᑯᓰᐅᑖᐸᓂᔫ. ᒨᓀᔮᐦᐦᒡ ᒫᒃ ᒌ ᐃᑎᔑᐦᐧᐋᑲᓅ ᑳᐱᒥᐦᔮᒪᑲᐦᐦᒡ ᐁᒌ ᐴᔑᐦᐧᐋᑲᓅᑦ.

ᓇᒧᐃ ᐅᐦᒌ ᒥᐧᔮᔫ ᐊᓂᔫ ᐅᔅᑳᑦ. ᑯᐧᑖᔅᒡ ᐲᓯᒼ ᒌ ᑯᒋᐦᑖᔫᐦ ᓂᑐᐦᑯᐃᓐᐦ ᒉᒌ ᐧᐄᒋᐦᐄᑯᑦ

CRACK !

Une douleur aiguë et familière fusa tout le long de sa bonne jambe. Il s'était cassé le genou. Son bon genou. Il n'aurait pas pu être moins chanceux.

Les médecins de la clinique l'envoyèrent en ambulance à l'hôpital de Chibougamau où un chirurgien fixa une plaque à la perceuse dans le genou pour le stabiliser, afin que Jack puisse guérir correctement. Puis défilèrent des semaines d'exercice et de rééducation, mais assez vite la bonne jambe au genou cassé guérit.

L'autre jambe, celle qui avait été cassée dans l'accident de voiture, continuait à le faire souffrir. Un soir, après le dîner, Jack commença à débiter du charabia à sa mère. Elle le regarda de près, droit dans les yeux – et appela une ambulance. Les médecins de la clinique firent transporter Jack par avion à Montréal.

La jambe de Jack ne guérissait pas. Pendant six mois, les médecins avaient

CRACK!

A sharp familiar pain shot through his good leg. He had busted his knee. The good one. Of all the dumb luck.

The clinic doctors sent him in an ambulance to the hospital in Chibougamau where a surgeon drilled a plate into the knee to stabilize it so Jack could heal properly. Then came weeks of exercise and rehabilitation, but soon enough the good leg with the busted knee healed.

The other leg, the one broken in the car accident, continued to hurt. One evening, after dinner, Jack began speaking gibberish to his Mom. She looked at him closely, right in the eye – and then called the ambulance. The doctors at the clinic had Jack airlifted to Montréal.

Jack's leg wasn't healing. For six months now, the doctors had tried but the

ᐧᐄᒋᐦᐄᑯᑦ ᓂᑐᐦᑯᔨᓐᐦ ᐊᔮᐱᒡ ᒌᐦ ᐊᑎ ᒫᔮᑎᓂᔨᐤ ᐊᓂᔮ ᐅᔅᑳᑦ᙮ ᐱᔥᒡ ᐊᓂᑎᐦ ᔖᔥ ᓈᔥᑎᔨᒡ ᓂᒥ ᐅᐦᒋ ᐃᐦᑖᔨᐤᐦ ᐅᔑᑮᐦ, ᑭᔮᐦ ᒧᔖ ᒌᐦ ᓅᑯᓂᔨᐤ ᐅᔅᑭᓐ ᐊᓂᑎᐦ ᑳᐦ ᓈᐧᑖᐱᔨᔨᒡ ᑳ ᐅᔑᑯᔑᐦᒃ᙮

ᓈᔥᒡ ᐋᐦ ᒌᐦ ᒫᑯᐦᐄᑯᑦ ᐋᐦ ᐋᐦᑯᓯᑦ᙮ ᐊᐧᑳᑎᑯᑦ ᒑᒃ ᐊᓂᔮᐦ ᓂᑐᐦᑯᔨᓐᐦ, “ᑖᐹ ᒋᑭ ᒋᐦ ᒥᐧᔮᐤ ᔖᔥ ᒋᔅᑳᑦ, ᐄᔑᓈᑯᓐ ᒐ ᒌᐦ ᒥᓂᔑᑭᓂᐧᐃᒡ”᙮ ᑯᐃᔅᒄ ᒌᐦ ᐊᔨᒥᐦᐄᑰ ᑭᔮᐦ ᒌᐦ ᒋᔅᑎᒫᒑᔨᒥᑰ᙮ ᓂᒧᐃ ᐅᐦᒋ ᑯᔥᑯᐦᑎᐧᐋᐤ ᒑᒃ ᑭᔮᐦ ᑏᐧᐋᐦᒡ ᒌᐦ ᓂᐦᐋᔨᐦᑎᒻ᙮

ᑳᐦ ᐹᔨᑯᑎᐧᐃᔥᑖᔨᒡ ᔖᔥ ᒌᐦ ᒥᓂᔑᑭᓂᐧᐃᔨᐤ ᐊᓂᔮ ᐅᔅᑳᑦ, ᐊᓂᑎᐦ ᓃᐦᑖᐦᒡ ᐅᐦᒋᑯᓂᐦᒡ᙮

ᑳᐦ ᒌᔑ ᒥᓂᔑᑭᓂᐧᐃᐧᐃᔨᒡ ᒫᒃ ᐊᓂᔮ ᐅᔅᑳᑦ, ᐹᔨᑯᑎᐧᐃᔥᑖᐤᐦ ᒌᐦ ᐃᐦᑖᐤ ᒑᒃ ᐊᓂᑖᐦ ᓈᔥᒡ ᐃᔮᐧᑳᐦ ᐋᐦ ᓈᓈᑭᒋᐦᐋᑭᓂᐧᐃᑦ ᐊᐧᐋᓐ ᐋᐦ ᐄᐦᑎᔮᑭᓂᐧᐃᑦ ᐋᐦ ᐱᔥᒑᔨᒡ᙮ ᐹᔨᐧᑳᐤ ᐋᐦ ᒌᐦᔑᑳᔨᐤ ᓈᔥᑎᔨᒡ ᓂᒥ ᐋᐦᒋᐱᔨᔨᐤ ᐊᓂᔮᐦ ᐋᐦ ᒥᓯᓂᐦᐄᒑᐱᔨᔨᒡ ᐋᐦ ᐄᔅᐱᔨᔨᒡ ᐊᐧᐋᓐ ᐅᑖᐃᐦ, ᓈᔥᑎᔨᒡ ᒋᐱᐦᒋᐱᔨᔨᐤ ᐧᒫᐦᒡ ᐊᓂᑖᐦ ᐊᐧᐋᓐ ᐋᑳ ᔖᔥ ᐱᒫᑎᓰᑦ᙮

ᐋᑯᑎᐦ ᐊᓂᑎᐦ ᐹᔓᒡ ᓂᐹᐧᐃᓂᐦᒡ ᑳᐦ ᓃᐳᐧᐃᔨᒡ ᐦ ᐅᑳᐧᐄᐦ ᐊᓂᔮ ᑳ ᐄᔅᐱᔨᒡ, ᒥᒄ ᐄᔑ ᐅᑎᑖᒥᐦᐧᑳᐦᐅᑰ ᔫᐦᒃ ᐊᓂᔮᐦ ᐅᑳᐧᐄᐦ: “ᑳ ᐧᐃᔥᑦ ᐧᐋᐦᐋᔨᐦᑎᐦ ᒌᒃ,” ᓈᔥᒡ ᐋᐦ ᒋᐧᔖᐧᐋᐦᑮᐦᑖᑯᑦ ᑭᔮᐦ ᒦᓐ ᔫᐦᒃ

ᒥᒄ ᒫᒃ ᔮᐸᒡ ᐁᑯᓐ ᑳᒌ ᐃᔅᐸᔨᓂᔨᒡ ᒦᓐ ᐁ ᐊᑎ ᒥᔫᓂᔨᒡ ᒫᓐᐦ᙮ ᒌ ᐃᐦᑕᑯᓂᔫ ᑲᔦ ᐊᓂᑕ ᓵᔅ ᐁᑳ ᒉᒋᒻ ᐧᐄᔮᓯᓂᔨᒡ, ᒥᒍᓐ ᐁ ᑰᑯᓂᔨᒡ ᐊᓂᔫ ᐅᔅᑳᑎᑲᓐ ᐊᓂᑕ ᑲ ᓈᐧᑖᐦᑎᓂᔨᒡ ᐊᓂᔫ ᐅᔅᑳᑦ᙮ ᑖᐧᐯ ᒌ ᐧᐄᓯᒉᔨᐦᑕᒥᐦᐄᑰ ᐊᓂᔫ ᐅᔅᑳᑦ᙮

ᓂᑐᐧᐁᔨᐦᑖᑯᓐ ᐁᑯᔥ ᒉᒌ ᒪᓂᔑᑲᓅᐦᒡ ᒋᔅᑳᑦ, ᒌ ᐄᑎᑰ ᓂᑐᐦᑯᐃᓐᐦ᙮ ᒋᔮᒻ ᒌ ᐊᔨᒥᐦᐄᑰ ᐅᔫ ᐧᐋᐦᑕᒫᑯᑦ᙮ ᒌ ᑯᔥᑯᐸᔫ ᑮᐸ ᐅᔫ ᐱᔦᐦᑕᐦᒃ ᑲ ᓇᓈᒥᔅᐧᑫᔨᑦ ᐁ ᓇᔅᑯᒧᑦ ᐅᔫ ᒉᒌ ᐃᐦᑑᑐᐧᐋᑲᓅᑦ᙮

ᒦᓐ ᑳ ᑑᔥᑌᔨᒡ ᓵᔅ ᓇᒧᐃ ᐅᐦᒋ ᐃᐦᑕᑯᓂᔫ ᐊᓂᔫ ᐅᔅᑳᑦ, ᓃᐦᑖᐦᒡ ᐅᐦᒋᑯᓂᐦᒡ ᐁᒌ ᒪᓂᔑᑲᓄᔨᒡ᙮

ᑳ ᐃᔅᐧᑳᒋᒥᔑᑲᓄᔨᒡ ᐅᔅᑳᑦ ᒌᒃ, ᐯᔭᑯᑑᔥᑌᐤᐦ ᒌ ᐃᐦᑖᐤ ᐋᐦᑯᔩᐅᑲᒥᑯᐦᒡ ᐊᓂᑌ ᔮᐧᑳᐤ ᓂᔮᓈᑲᒋᐦᐋᑲᓅᑦ ᐊᐧᐁᓐ ᐁ ᐋᐦᑯᓯᑦ ᐁᑯᑌ ᐄᑌᐦᒉ ᑳ ᑲᓇᐧᐁᔨᒫᑲᓅᑦ᙮ ᐁᒄ ᒫᒃ ᐯᔭᐧᑳᐤ ᐊᓂᔫ ᑳᒪᓯᓈᐅᔥᑌᐸᔨᔑᔨᒡ ᐊᓂᑕᐦ ᐧᐁᐦᒋ ᓈᓈᑲᒋᐦᑖᑲᓅᔫ ᐊᐧᐁᓐ ᐅᑌᐦᐄᐦ, ᒌ ᓅᑯᓂᔫ ᐁ ᒋᐱᐦᒋᐸᔨᒡ ᐅᑌᐦᐃ, ᒋᔑᓀ ᐁ ᒋᔅᑑᒪᑲᓂᔨᒡ, ᒥᒋᐦᐱᓐ ᐱᔦᐦᑖᑯᐦᒡ ᐊᓐ ᐁᑯᑦ ᐧᐁᐦᒋ ᒋᔅᑫᔨᑖᑲᓅᐦᒡ ᐁᑳ ᓵᔅ ᐃᐦᑖᑦ ᐊᓐ ᐊᐧᐁᓐ᙮

ᐁᑯᑦ ᑳ ᓃᐳᔨᒡ ᐅᑳᐧᐄ ᐅᔫ ᑳ ᐃᔅᐸᔨᑦ ᒌᒃ, ᔫᐦᒃ ᑳ ᐅᑖᒥᐦᐧᑫᐦᐧᐋᑦ ᐊᓂᔫ ᐅᑯᓴ᙮ “ᐁᑯᓐ ᐃᔥᐱᔥ ᒌᔅᐧᑫᐦᑳᓯ, ᒌᒃ”, ᒌᔑ ᐋᔥᐧᑳᑌᐤ, ᐁᒄ ᒦᓐ ᑳ ᐅᑖᒥᐦᐧᑫᐦᐧᐋᑦ᙮ “ᐁᑳᐧᐄ ᓇᑲᔑᐦ, ᓂᑲ ᒥᔅᑕ ᒋᔑᐧᐋᓯᓐ ᒫᒌᔨᓀ”, ᒌᔑ ᐋᔥᐧᑫᐤ᙮

essayé, mais l'infection continuait de lui manger la jambe. À certains endroits, la chair avait complètement disparu et on pouvait voir l'os à nu qui avait été brisé dans l'accident de voiture. La douleur était incroyable.

infection continued to eat his leg. In some areas, the flesh was completely gone, and you could see the naked bone that had been broken in the car accident. The pain was unbelievable.

« Nous allons devoir amputer », dit finalement le médecin. Il était direct et gentil tout à la fois. Jack n'était pas surpris et acquiesça son consentement.

"We're going to have to amputate," the doctor finally said. He was frank and kind all at once. Jack wasn't surprised and nodded his consent.

Une semaine plus tard, la partie inférieure de sa jambe avait disparu, coupée en dessous du genou.

A week later his lower leg was gone, cut off below the knee.

Après cette amputation, Jack passa une semaine à l'hôpital, dans l'unité de soins intensifs. Un jour, la machine branchée sur son cœur émit soudainement le bip continu d'une personne qui n'est plus en vie.

After that amputation surgery, Jack spent a week in the hospital in the Intensive Care Unit. One day, the machine hooked up to his heart flatlined and sounded the continual beep of someone no longer alive.

La mère de Jack, qui se tenait à côté du lit lorsque cela se produisit, le gifla fort : « Arrête de faire l'imbécile, Jack, cria-t-elle et le gifla de nouveau. Tu ferais mieux de revenir ou je vais être assez fâchée

Jack's mother was standing there beside the bed when it happened and she slapped him hard: "Stop fooling around, Jack," she shouted and slapped him again. "You better come back or I'm gonna be so

ᐧᐋᑎᑖᒥᐦᐧᑳᐦᐅᑯᑦ᙮ "ᐋᑳᐧᐄ ᒫᔥᒋᐤ ᒫᒌᐦ, ᓈᔥᑖᐧᐹᐦ ᒋᑭ ᒋᔑᐧᐋᐦᐄᓐ᙮"

ᐱᔮᐱᐦᑖᔨᒡᐦ ᓂᑐᐦᑯᔨᓐᐦ ᑮᔮᐦ ᓂᑐᐦᑯᔨᓂᔅᐧᑳᐤᐦ ᒑᔅᒑᔨᐦᑎᒥᔨᒡᐦ ᐋᐦ ᒋᐱᐦᒋᐱᔨᔨᒡ ᒑᐧᑳᔨᐤ᙮ ᑏᐧᐋᐦᒡ ᒋᔅᒑᔨᑎᒻ ᒑᒃ ᔮᔨᑖ ᑮᔮᐦ ᑏᐧᐋᐦᒡ ᒑ ᓈᑭᔑᒋᐦᐋᑦ ᐅᑳᐧᐄᐦ᙮ ᒑᒃ ᒦᓐ ᐱᔮᐱᔨᔨᒡ ᐋᐦ ᐋᐦᒋᐱᔨᔨᒡ ᐅᑖᐃᐦ, ᐋᑎ ᒌᐧᐋᐱᔨᐦᐧᐃᔨᒡᐦ ᐊᓂᔮᐦ ᓂᑐᐦᑯᔨᓈᐱᑎᓰᓯᐤᐦ, ᑮᔮᐦ ᐧᐋᑎᒥᔨᒡᐦ ᐊᓂᔮ ᑳ ᒋᐱᐦᐧᑖᐧᐋᐱᔨᔨᒡ᙮

ᐊᑎᑎᐤ ᒫᒃ ᑳ ᐋᑎ ᒥᔪᐱᒫᑎᓰᑦ ᒑᒃ, ᑳ ᒥᔮᑭᓂᐧᐃᑦ ᒥᔅᑳᑎᐦᑳᔨᐤ᙮ ᐊᓂᔮ ᒫᒃ ᑳ ᒥᔮᑭᓂᐧᐃᑦ ᐧᒫᐦᒡ ᐊᓂᑖᐦ ᐅᑖᐹᓈᔅᑯᐦ ᐋᐦ ᐅᑎᓂᒫᑦ ᐊᐧᐋᓐ ᐋᑯᑖᐦ ᐋᔑᓈᑯᐦᒡ᙮ ᐋᐦ ᐧᐋᐦᑎᐦᒡ ᒋᑭ ᒌᐦ ᐅᑎᓈᓐ ᑮᔮᐦ ᒫᒃ ᓈᔥᒡ ᐋᐦ ᒥᐧᔮᒡ᙮ ᐊᓂᔮ ᒫᒃ ᑳ ᒥᔮᑭᓂᐧᐃᑦ ᒑᒃ ᓂᒧᐃ ᓈᔥᒡ ᐅᐦᒋ ᒥᐧᔮᔨᐤ᙮ ᓈᔥᒡ ᐋᐦ ᒌᐦ ᐧᐃᔥᑎᐧᐃᔥᑳᑯᑦ, ᐋᐦ ᐹᐱᑯᐦᐅᑯᑦ, ᑮᔮᐦ ᓈᔥᒡ ᐋᐦ ᒌᐦ ᐧᐃᔥᑎᐧᐃᔥᑭᐦᒃ᙮ ᓂᒧᐃ ᑯᐃᔅᒄ ᐅᐦᒋ ᑖᐱᒧᔨᐤ = ᒥᒄ ᑳ ᔒᐱᐱᔨᔨᒡ ᒌᐦ ᐋᐱᑎᓂᔨᐤ ᐋᑳ ᒥᒄ ᒑ ᒌᐦ ᐄᔑ ᒥᓂᐱᔨᔨᒡ᙮ ᓂᔮᓂᑯᑑᓐᐦ ᑳ ᒌ ᒥᓂᐱᔨᔨᒡ ᑮᔮᐦ ᓈᔥᒡ ᑳ ᒌ ᐧᐃᔥᑎᐧᐃᔥᑭᐦᒃ ᑮᔮᐦ ᑳ ᒌ ᒥᒥᔅᑳᓯᓂᐧᐋᑭᓂᐧᐃᑦ ᒑᒃ ᐅᔮ ᐋᓂᔨᒡᐦ᙮ ᐊᓂᑖᐦ ᑳ ᒌ ᐄᔑ ᑭᓂᐧᐋᐱᐦᑎᐦᒃ, ᐋᑯᑎᐦ ᑳ ᒌ ᐧᐋᐱᐦᑎᐦᒃ ᓈᔥᒡ ᓂᑎᐧᐄ ᐋᐦ ᐄᑎᒧᔨᒡ ᐊᓂᔮ ᐅᔅᑳᑦ᙮ ᒌᐦ ᐧᔔᐧᑳᔨᒧᐦᐄᑰ᙮ ᐋᔪᐧᐃᒄ ᒫᒃ ᐊᓂᔮ ᒥᔅᑳᑎᐦᑳᓂᔨᐤ ᑳ ᒥᔮᑭᓂᐧᐃᑦ ᑮᔮᐦ ᑳ ᐅᐦᒋ ᑎᐱᐦᐄᑭᓂᐧᐃᐧᐃᔨᒡ ᐊᓂᑖᐦ ᐅᐦᒋ ᐄᔨᔨᐤ ᓂᑐᐦᑯᔨᓈᐱᑎᓰᐧᐃᓂᐦᒡ᙮ ᑳᐦ ᑯᒋᔥᑖᑦ ᑭᔨᐧᐹ ᑯᐃᔅᒄ ᒑ ᐧᐄᐦ ᐄᔑᓈᑯᐦᑖᑦ

ᐁᒄ ᐊᓂᒌ ᓂᑐᐦᑯᐃᓐ ᑲᔦ ᓂᑐᐦᑯᐃᓂᔅᐧᑫᐅᒡ ᑳ ᓈᒋᐸᐦᐧᑖᐧᑖᐤ ᐊᓂᔫ ᑳ ᐱᒥᐸᔨᔑᔨᒡ ᒥᑌᐦᐄᐦ ᐁᐧᐄ ᐧᐄᒋᔥᑖᑲᓅᐦᒡ ᒦᓐ ᑫᒌ ᐸᐦᑲᐦᐊᐦᒡ᙮ ᒌ ᒋᔥᑫᔨᐦᑕᒻ ᒫᒃ ᒑᒃ ᑫᒌ ᐱᔑᒋᐦᐋᑦ ᐅᑳᐧᐄ᙮ ᑳ ᐹᐸᔨᐦᑖᑲᓅᔨᒡ ᐊᓂᔫ ᒋᐹ ᐋᐸᑕᓂᔫ ᒦᓐ ᑫᒌ ᐸᐦᑲᐦᐊᓂᔨᒡ ᐅᐦᑌᐦᐄ ᓵᔅ ᑳᐤ ᒌ ᒥᔫᐸᔨᓂᔫ ᐊᓂᔫ ᐅᑌᐦᐄ ᐁᒄ ᑳᐤ ᑳ ᐧᐄᐧᐄᐦᑕᑖᐧᑖᐤ ᐊᓂᒌ ᓂᑐᐦᑯᐃᓂᒡ ᑲᔦ ᓂᑐᐦᑯᐃᓂᔅᐧᑫᐅᒡ ᐊᓂᔫ ᒋᐹ ᐋᐸᒋᐦᑖᐅᒡ᙮

ᐧᐁᑖᒡ ᒫᒃ ᒌ ᐊᑎ ᒥᐧᔮᔫ ᐅᔅᑳᑦ, ᐁᒄ ᑳ ᑯᒋᔥᑲᒧᑎᔮᑲᓅᑦ ᒥᔅᑳᑎᐦᑳᓂᔫ᙮ ᒧᐧᐁᐦᒡ ᒫᒃ ᐅᒑᐹᓂᔥ ᐁᐧᐄ ᐅᑎᓂᑲᓅᐦᒡ ᐃᑌᔮᐦᑖᑯᓐ ᒥᔅᑳᑎᐦᑳᓐ ᐁᐧᐄ ᐅᑎᓂᑲᓅᐦᒡ᙮ ᐧᐁᐦᑕᒋᐦᑖᑯᓐᐦ ᐸᔅᒡ ᐁᒄ ᑯᑕᒃ ᐁ ᐧᔔᓕᔮᐅᐦᐧᑳᐤ᙮ ᐊᓂᔫ ᒥᔅᑳᑎᐦᑳᓂᔫ ᑳ ᑯᒋᔥᑲᒧᑎᔮᑲᓅᑦ ᓇᒧᐃ ᐅᐦᒋ ᐧᔔᓕᔮᐅᓂᔫ᙮ ᒌᐧᐄ ᐸᑲᐦᐆᑰ ᐊᓂᔫ ᒥᔅᑳᑎᐦᑳᓂᔫ ᐊᓂᑕ ᑳ ᐅᐦᒋ ᒋᒥᔑᑲᓅᔨᒡ ᐊᓂᔫ ᐅᔅᑳᑦ᙮ ᓇᒧᐃ ᓇᐦᐋᐤ ᐅᐦᒋ ᑖᐱᐦᑎᓂᔫ = ᐹᑎᔅ ᒌ ᐋᔅᐸᐦᐄᑲᓅᔫ ᐁᑳ ᑫᒌ ᐋᐦᒋᐸᔨᔨᒡ᙮ ᓂᔮᓂᑯᑌᐦᒡ ᒌ ᐅᑖᐯᐸᔨᐦᑖᐤ ᒫᒃ ᓂᑐᐧᐄᓐ ᒌ ᐃᑕᑯᑌᔫ ᐁᒄ ᓈᔅᒡ ᑳᒌ ᑲᓇᐧᐋᐸᒥᑯᑦ ᐊᐧᐁᔫᐦ᙮ ᐅᔅᑳᑦ ᑮᐹ ᐊᓂᔫ ᑳ ᑲᓇᐧᐋᐸᐦᑖᑲᓅᔨᒡ ᓈᔅᒡ ᐁᑳ ᒨᔮᒻ ᐃᔑᓈᑯᓂᔨᒡ᙮ ᒌᐧᐃ ᐧᔔᐧᑫᔨᒥᐦᐄᑰ ᐅᔫ ᐁ ᐃᔅᐸᔨᑦ᙮ ᐁᐅᒄ ᑮᐹ ᐅᔫ ᒥᔅᑳᑎᐦᑲᓂᔫ ᑳ ᒦᔮᑲᓅᑦ ᐊᓂᑌ ᐅᐦᒋ ᒥᔫᐱᒫᑎᓰᐧᐃᓐ ᐁ ᐅᐦᒋ ᓇᓈᑲᒋᐦᑖᑲᓅᒡ᙮ ᑳ ᑯᒋᐦᑖᑦ ᑳᐤ ᑫᒌ ᒥᔫᒧᐦᑖᑦ ᐁᒄ ᑳᒌ ᒌᐧᐁᑦ᙮ ᒌ ᓂᑑ ᐋᐸᓯᑑ ᐁᒄ ᐃᔅᑯᑕᒃ ᑳ ᐃᔅᐧᑳᐤ ᐋᐸᑎᓯᑦ ᑳᒌ ᓂᑑ ᐧᐄᒋᒥᓂᐦᐧᑫᒫᑦ ᐅᐧᐄᒉᐧᐋᑲᓐᐦ᙮

contre toi ! »

Les médecins et les infirmières s'empressèrent vers le chariot de réanimation. Toutefois, Jack savait qu'il ne fallait pas désobéir à sa mère. Son cœur battait à nouveau régulièrement lorsque le chariot arriva et le personnel de l'hôpital fit demi-tour, emportant le chariot de réanimation avec eux.

Une fois que Jack eut guéri davantage, les médecins lui installèrent une jambe artificielle, une prothèse. Les prothèses, cependant, sont un peu comme les voitures. On peut les acheter à bon marché ou de haute gamme. La nouvelle jambe de Jack n'était pas la meilleure des prothèses. Elle frottait sur le moignon. Elle n'était pas bien ajustée. Elle ne pouvait pas être verrouillée en place. Le tout était maintenu en place par une seule feuille de caoutchouc au niveau du moignon, de sorte qu'elle glissait trop facilement. Parfois, elle glissait ou se déplaçait à un angle bizarre de sorte que les gens regardaient Jack bizarrement. Il jetait alors un coup d'œil vers le bas et voyait sa jambe qui partait frénétiquement dans toutes les directions. C'était assez embarrassant. Toutefois,

mad at you!"

The doctors and nurses went running for the crash cart. Jack knew better than to disobey his mom, though. His heart machine was beating regularly again by the time the cart arrived, and the hospital staff turned right around, taking the crash cart with them.

After Jack had healed further, the doctors fitted him with an artificial leg, a prosthesis. Prostheses, though, are a little bit like cars. You can buy them cheaply made or you can buy them well made. Jack's new leg wasn't the best prosthesis. It rubbed at the stump. It didn't fit properly. It couldn't be locked into place – the whole thing was held in place by a single sheet of rubber at the stump so it would slip off too easily. Sometimes it would drag or slip out of place at a weird angle and people would look at Jack strangely. He would glance down then and see his leg, madly off in all directions. Kind of embarrassing. But it was the prosthesis that the Cree Board of Health paid for. He attached it to his stump as best he could and went back home. Back to work and to beers after work with the boys.

ᑮᔮᐦ ᒦᓐ ᑳ ᐋᑎ ᒌᐧᐋᑦ᙮ ᒦᓐ ᑳ ᒋᔅᑖᐱᑎᓰᑦ
ᑮᔮᐦ ᒦᓐ ᑳᐦ ᒋᔥᒌᑦ ᐋᐦ ᒥᓂᐦᐧᑳᑦ ᐅᐧᐄᒑᐧᐋᑮᓐᐦ
ᐋᐦ ᐧᐄᒋᒥᓂᐦᐧᑳᒫᑦ᙮

ᓈᔥᒡ ᒫᒃ ᐹᑎᒫᐦ ᐊᓂᔮ ᑳ ᐄᔥᐱᔑ ᒌᐧᐋᒡ,
ᒫᐧᑳᒡ ᒌᐦ ᐧᐄᒋᒦᒋᓯᒫᐤ ᒑᒃ ᐅᑳᐧᐄᐦ᙮

ᐊᐧᑳᑖᑦ, "ᓈᑳ, ᐊᓂᑖᐦ ᒫᒃ ᐧᒫᓐᑎᓅᐧᔮᑦ ᑳ
ᐃᐦᑖᔨᐦᒄ ᐊᓂᑖᐦ ᓂᐹᐅᑭᒥᑯᐦᒡ ᑳ ᐃᐦᑖᔮᐦᒄ,
ᓈᔥᒡ ᐋᐦ ᒌᐦ ᒥᐧᔮᔑᒡ ᑮᔮᐦ ᓈᔥᒡ ᐋᐦ ᒌᐦ
ᐋᔨᒥᒋᔥᑖᑯᐦᒡ᙮ ᓈᔥᒡ ᑳ ᒥᔖᒡ ᐋᐦ ᐧᐋᐹᒡ
ᓂᐹᐧᐃᓐ ᑮᔮᐦ ᐊᓂᐦᐄ ᐧᐋᐳᔮᓐᐦ ᑳ ᐧᐋᐹᒡᐦ
ᑮᔮᐦ ᐊᓂᐦᐄ ᐋᑯᔮᑭᐦᐄᑭᓐᐦ ᐋᐦ ᐧᐋᐧᐋᐹᔥᑎᔑᒡᐦ
ᐊᓂᑖᐦ ᐋᐦ ᐹᒋ ᔫᑎᔑᒡ ᑮᔮᐦ ᓈᔥᒡ ᐋᐦ ᒌᐦ
ᐄᔥᐹᒡ ᐊᓂᑖᐦ ᐄᔥᐱᒥᐦᒡ ᐋᐦ ᐄᑖᐱᓈᓂᐧᐃᒡ
ᐊᓐ ᓂᐹᐅᑭᒥᒄ᙮ ᐋᐦ ᒌᐦ ᐹᐦᑖᑯᓯᒡ ᐊᐧᐋᓂᒌ
ᐊᓂᑎᐦ ᐧᐃᔨᐧᐄᑎᒥᐦᒡ ᐋᐦ ᒥᐧᑖᔨᒥᒡ ᒧᔮᒻ
ᐊᓂᑖᐦ ᓈᔥᒡ ᐋᐦ ᒧᒋᒑᔨᐦᑎᐦᒡ ᐦ ᐊᓂᑖ ᐋᐦ
ᐱᒧᐦᑖᓂᐧᐃᐧᐄᔨᒡ᙮ ᒑᒄ ᓂᐹᐅᑭᒥᒄ ᐊᓐ᙮ ᑖᓂᑖᐦ
ᐧᐋᐦᒋ ᒌᐦ ᑎᐱᐦᐋᒥᐦᒄ᙮"

ᓈᔥᒡ ᐋᐦ ᑯᔥᑯᒫᑦ ᐊᓂᔮᐦ ᐅᑳᐧᐄᐦ, ᐊᐧᑳᑎᑯᑦ,
"ᒑᒃ, ᑖᐹ ᑰᐦᒋᔥᑖᓐ ᐊᓂᑖᐦ ᓂᐹᐅᑭᒥᑯᐦᒡ᙮ ᒥᒄ
ᐊᓂᑖᐦ ᐋᐦᑯᓰᐅᑭᒥᑯᐦᒡ ᐊᔥᒌᐦ ᐃᐦᑖᓐ, ᐋᑯᐦ
ᓃᔨ ᐊᓂᑖᐦ ᓂᐹᐅᑭᒥᑯᐦᒡ ᑳ ᐃᐦᑖᔮᓐ᙮ ᓂᒧᐃ
ᒥᒄ ᐅᐦᒋ ᐋᔨᒥᒋᔥᑖᑯᓐ ᑮᔮᐦ ᐅᐦᒋ ᐄᔥᐱᔑ
ᒥᐧᔮᐤ᙮"

"ᓂᒋᔅᒋᓯᓐ ᐧᐋᔥ", ᐄᑖᐤ, "ᒥᑐᓐ ᑯᐃᔅᑯ
ᓂᒋᔅᒋᓰᑎᑖᓐ" "ᓂᐧᐹᔨᒻ, ᐄᑎᑰ, ᐧᐋᔥ ᐊᓐ

ᐯᔭᐧᑳᐤ, ᐃᔅᑯᑕᒃ ᑳᐤ ᐁ ᒌᐧᐁᑦ ᒑᒃ, ᒌ
ᐧᐄᒋᒦᒋᓰᒣᐤ ᐅᑳᐧᐄ ᐁ ᐋᐱᐦᑖᒌᔑᑳᔮᒡ᙮

ᑳ ᐄᑖᑦ ᐊᓂᔮ ᐅᑳᐧᐄ, "ᒫᒫ, ᒧᓕᔮᐦᒡ ᒫ ᑳ
ᐃᐦᑖᔨᐦᒄ ᓂᐯᐅᑲᒥᑯᐦᒡ ᒋᒌ ᐃᐦᑖᓈᓅ᙮ ᒌ
ᔖᓕᔮᐅᓐ ᐊᓂᑕ ᑳ ᓂᐹᔨᐦᒄ ᑲᔦ ᒌ ᒥᐧᔮᔖ᙮
ᒌ ᐧᐋᐹᔖ ᒋ ᓂᐯᐧᐃᓂᓅ, ᑲᔦ ᐧᐋᐳᔮᓐᐦ ᒌ
ᐧᐋᐹᐤ, ᑲᔦ ᐊᓂᐦᐄᐦ ᐋᑰᔦᑲᐦᐄᑲᓐᐦ ᒌ ᐧᐋᐹᐤ
ᒣᒋᒻ ᐊᓂᑌ ᐃᔅᐱᒥᐦᒡ ᒌ ᐧᐋᐹᐤ᙮ ᒌ ᐯᐦᑖᑯᓰᒡ
ᐊᐧᐁᓂᒌ ᐊᓂᑕ ᐧᐄᐧᐄᑎᒥᐦᒡ ᐁ ᒪᐧᑌ ᐊᔨᒥᐧᑖᐤ᙮
ᒧᔮᒻ ᐁ ᒥᓂᐦᐧᑳᓅᒡ ᒌ ᐃᑎᐦᑖᑯᓐ᙮ ᑖᓐ ᑳ
ᐃᔑᓂᐦᑲᑌᒡ ᐊᓂᑕ ᑳ ᓂᐹᔨᐦᒄ᙮ ᑖᓂᑌ ᑳ ᐅᐦᒋ
ᒌᔫᐦᑲᒥᐦᒄ ᐊᓂᑕ ᑳ ᐃᐦᑖᔨᐦᒄ"᙮

ᑳ ᑲᓇᐧᐋᐸᒥᑯᑦ ᐅᑳᐧᐄ ᑳ ᐄᑎᑯᑦ, "ᒑᒃ, ᓇᒧᐃ
ᓂᐯᐅᑲᒥᑯᐦᒡ ᑰᐦᒋ ᐃᐦᑖᓈᓅ᙮ ᐋᐦᑯᓰᐅᑲᒥᑯᐦᒡ
ᒋᒌ ᐃᐦᑖᓐ ᒌᔭ ᐁᑯ ᓃ ᓂᐯᐅᑲᒥᑯᐦᒡ ᑳ
ᐃᐦᑖᔮᓐ᙮ ᓇᒧᐃ ᒫᒃ ᒥᒍᓐ ᐅᐦᒋ ᐃᔑᓈᑯᓐ ᐊᓐ
ᓂᓂᐯᐅᑲᒥᒄ ᐊᓂᑕ ᑳ ᓂᐹᔮᓐ"᙮

ᐁᑯ ᑳ ᐃᐧᑌᑦ ᒑᒃ, "ᓂᒋᔅᒋᓯᓐ ᐧᐁᓯᓐ,
ᓂᒣᔥᑎᓈᐦᐅᓐ ᐁᑯᑦ ᐊᓂᑕ ᑳ ᐃᐦᑖᔨᐦᒄ"᙮

il s'agissait de la prothèse pour laquelle le Conseil cri de la santé avait payé. Il l'attachait à son moignon du mieux possible et rentrait chez lui. Retour au travail et aux bières après le travail avec les *chums*.

Quelques semaines plus tard, Jack déjeunait avec sa mère.

« Maman, quand nous étions à Montréal, nous avons séjournés dans une chambre d'hôtel. Une très belle chambre, très chère. Avec un grand lit blanc et des draps blancs et des rideaux blancs que la brise faisait voler un peu vers l'intérieur et un haut plafond blanc. Les gens parlaient à l'extérieur de la chambre. Comme s'ils faisaient la fête dans le couloir. Quel était cet hôtel ? Comment pouvions-nous nous permettre de nous l'offrir ? »

Elle le regarda un peu bizarrement et lui dit : « Jack, tu n'as jamais séjourné dans un hôtel. Tu étais à l'hôpital et j'ai séjourné à l'hôtel. Mon hôtel n'était *pas du tout* comme ça ».

« Mais je m'en souviens, dit-il. J'en suis sûr ».

A few weeks later, Jack was having lunch with his mom.

"Mom, when we were in Montréal, we stayed in a hotel room. A really nice expensive room. With a big white bed and white sheets and white curtains that blew in a bit with the breeze and a high white ceiling. People were talking outside the room. Like they were having a party in the hallway. Which hotel was that? How could we afford it?"

She looked at him a little strangely, and said, "Jack, you never stayed in a hotel. You stayed in the hospital and I stayed in a hotel. My hotel wasn't *anything* like that."

"But I remember," he said. "I'm sure of it."

ᐊᔅᒌᐦ ᐆᓂᐱᒫᑎᓰᓐ᙮ ᒌᐦ ᓅᑯᓐ ᐊᓂᑎᐦ ᐋ̈ᑳ ᓈᔥᑎᔪᒡ ᐋᐦᒋᐱᔪᒡ ᐊᔥᑖᐃᐦ᙮ ᐊᔥᒌᐦ ᐅᑎᑖᒥᐦᐧᑳᐦᐅᑎᓐ ᑭᔫᐦ ᐊᔥᒌᐦ ᒋᐧᔔᐧᐋᐦᑭᐦᑖᑎᓐ ᒑ ᐹᒋ ᒌᐧᐋᔪᓐ᙮ ᒫᔫᐤ ᒫᒃ ᐊᔥᒌᐦ ᐃᐦᑎᓐ ᑳ ᐹᒋ ᒌᐧᐋᔪᓐ, ᓈᔥᑖᐧᐹᐦ ᒋᐱᐦᒌᐦ ᒋᔑᐧᐋᐦᐄᓐ ᐋ̈ᑳ ᐅᐦᒋ ᐹᒋ ᒌᐧᐋᔪᓐ᙮”

ᐊᓂᔫ ᒫᒃ ᓂᐹᐅᑭᒥᑯᔪᐤ ᑭᔪᐧᐹ ᑳᐦ ᐃᐦᑎᑯᓂᔪᒡ, ᒥᒄ ᒫᒃ ᓂᒥᔫᐅᑎᐦ ᐅᑎᐦ ᓈᐦᐊᐤ ᐅᔫ ᐊᔅᒌᔪᐤ᙮

ᐄᔅᑯᑎᒃ ᒫᒃ ᑳ ᒌᔑᐦᑖᑦ ᒑᒃ ᐊᓂᔫ ᑳ ᐄᔑ ᓂᑎᐧᐋᔪᒫᑭᓂᐧᐃᑦ ᒐ ᐄᔑ ᔔᔔᐧᐄᑦ ᑭᔫᐦ ᐊᓂᔫ ᑳ ᐧᐄᐦ ᐄᔑ ᓂᑎᐧᐋᔪᒫᑭᓂᐧᐃᑦ ᒐ ᐄᔥᐱᔥ ᐃᔪᐧᐋᔑᑦ, ᑳᐦ ᐃᔫᔅᑭᐧᐄᑦ ᒦᓐ ᒐ ᒋᔥᑖᐱᑎᓰᑦ᙮ ᐋᐦᐧᒫᔫᐦ ᒫᒃ ᒌᐦ ᒫᒌᑦ, ᑳ ᐹᒋ ᒥᐧᑖᐦᑖᑯᑦ ᐊᓂᔫ ᐅᒋᒫᒻᐦ ᐊᓂᑖᐦ ᐧᐄᒋᐧᐋᐦᒡ᙮ ᐊᓂᔫ ᑳ ᐋᐱᒋᐦᐄᑯᑦ ᓂᒧᐃ ᐅᐦᒋ ᓂᑎᐧᐋᔪᒥᑰ ᐊᓂᔫ ᒦᓐ ᒐ ᐄᑖᐱᑎᓰᑦ ᐊᓂᑖᐦ ᐧᐃᔪᐧᐄᑎᒥᐦᒡ ᐋᐦ ᒌᐦ ᐋᐱᑎᓰᑦ, ᐄᑎᑰ ᐊᓂᔫᐦ ᐅᒋᒫᒻᐦ᙮ ᐊᓂᔫ ᒫᒃ ᑳ ᐅᔥᑳᔪᒡ ᐅᔅᑳᑎᐦᑳᓐ, ᒌᐦ ᒋᔅᒑᔪᐦᑎᒥᔪᐤᐦ ᒦᓐ ᑳᐤ ᒐ ᒌᐦ ᐃᐦᑐᑎᐦᒃ ᐊᓂᔫ ᐅᑖᐱᑎᓰᐧᐃᓐ, ᒨᔥ ᑭᔪᐧᐹ ᓈᔥᒡ ᐋᐦ ᒌᐦ ᒥᐧᔫᐱᑎᓰᑦ᙮ ᒌᐦ ᑯᔅᐱᓈᔪᐦᑎᒥᔪᐤᐦ ᒐ ᑎᐱᐦᐄᒐᔪᒡᐦ ᒥᔑᐤ ᐧᐃᔫᔥ ᐃᔪᐦᑎᒑ ᒐᒃ ᒫᐧᑳᒡ ᐋᐦ ᐋᐱᑎᓰᑦ ᐊᓂᑖᐦ ᐧᐃᔪᐧᐄᑎᒥᐦᒡ ᐅᐦᒋ ᐧᐄᔫᔅᐱᔪᔪᒐ ᐊᓂᔫ ᐅᔅᑳᑎᐦᑳᓐ᙮ ᓂᒧᐃ ᐅᐦᒋ ᓂᑎᐧᐋᔪᐦᑎᒧᒡ ᐊᓂᔫ ᒐ ᐄᔅᐱᔪᔪᒡ᙮ ᐋᑯᐦ ᑳ ᐄᑖᑭᓂᐧᐃᑦ ᒐᒃ ᐲᐦᑎᑭᒥᐦᒡ ᒐ ᐋᐱᑎᓰᑦ, ᐊᓂᑖᐦ ᒥᓯᓂᐦᐄᒑᐅᑭᒥᑯᐦᒡ᙮

“ᓂᑯᔥ, ᒋᒌ ᓂᐱᓐ ᐧᐁᔑᓐ᙮ ᒋᑌᐦᐄᐦ ᒌ ᒋᐱᐦᒋᐸᔮ᙮ ᒋᒌ ᐅᑕᑖᒍᐦᐧᑫᐦᐆᑎᓐ ᑲᔦ ᒋᒌ ᑌᐧᐹᑎᑎᓐ ᑳᐤ ᒦᓐ ᒉᒌ ᔦᐦᔦᔮᓐ᙮ ᐁᑳ ᑳᐤ ᐅᐦᒋ ᐱᒫᑎᓯᔮᓐ ᓅᐧᐊᒡ ᒋᐹ ᒋᔑᐧᐋᐦᐄᓐ”, ᒌ ᐄᑎᑰ ᐅᑳᐧᐄ᙮

ᐊᓂᔮ ᓂᐯᐅᑲᒥᑯᔮ ᑳ ᐋᔪᒎᑕᐦᒃ ᒑᒃ, ᓇᒧᐃ ᐅᑕ ᐊᔅᒌᐦᒡ ᐊᓂᔮ ᑳ ᐃᔑᓇᐦᒃ᙮

ᐃᔅᑯᑕᒃ ᒋᐦᒋᐧᐁ ᐁᑳ ᐅᐦᒋ ᓂᑐᐧᐁᔪᐦᑕᐦᒃ ᐁᑎᑑ ᒉᒌ ᓴᓵᐅᐸᔪᐦᐋᑲᓅᑦ ᑲᔦ ᓵᔅ ᐁᒌ ᐃᐦᑑᑐᐧᐋᑲᓅᑦ ᑖᓐ ᒋᐹ ᐃᐦᑑᑕᐧᐋᑲᓅ ᒉᒌ ᒥᔮᐸᔪᑦ, ᐁᒄ ᑳ ᐊᔦᔅᑲᐧᐄᔪᑦ ᒦᓐ ᑳᐤ ᒉᒌ ᓂᑑ ᐋᐸᑎᓯᑦ᙮ ᐁᑯᑦ ᒫᒃ ᐊᓂᑕ ᒉᐧᑳᒡ ᐅᒋᒫᒻ ᒌ ᑖᐦᑲᐱᐦᑫᓇᒫᑰ ᐊᓂᑌ ᐧᐄᒋᐦᒡ ᐁ ᐃᐦᑖᑦ᙮ ᑳ ᐧᐄᐦᑕᒫᑯᑦ ᐊᓂᔮ ᐅᒋᒫᒻ ᐁᑳ ᓂᑐᐧᐁᔪᐦᑖᑯᓯᑦ ᑳᐤ ᒉᒌ ᐋᐸᑎᓯᑦ ᐊᓂᔮ ᑲᒌ ᐄᑖᐸᑎᓯᑦ ᓂᑑᐦᐆᓂᔮ ᑲᔦ ᐁ ᐅᒋᐧᑳᒑᓄᔪᒡ ᑲᔦ ᐊᔅᒋᔮ ᐁ ᓇᓈᑲᒋᐦᑖᑦ᙮ ᒌ ᐅᔅᑳᔮ ᐅᔅᑳᑎᐦᑳᓐ, ᒌ ᑌᐯᔪᒎ ᒦᓐ ᑳᐤ ᒉᒌ ᓈᑕᐦᒃ ᐊᓂᔮ ᐅᑖᐸᑎᓯᐧᐃᓐ, ᒌ ᒋᔅᒉᔪᐦᑕᒥᔮ ᒫᒃ ᐊᓂᔮ ᑲᔦ ᒌ ᒋᔅᒉᔪᒥᑰ ᐁ ᒥᐧᔫᐸᑎᓯᑦ᙮ ᒥᒄ ᒫᒃ ᒌ ᓴᒋᓰᒡ ᒦᓐ ᐧᐃᔦᔅ ᒉᒌ ᐃᔅᐸᔪᔪᒡ ᒑᒃ ᒉᐧᑳᒡ ᐊᓂᐧᑌ ᓅᐦᒋᒦᐦᒡ ᐁ ᐋᐸᑎᓯᔪᒡ᙮ ᐧᐄᔪ ᐊᓐ ᑲᒻᐸᓃ ᒋᐸ ᒌᔒᐦᑲᒻ ᐃᓐᓯᕋᓐᔅ ᑫᒃ ᑫᐧᑳᔮ ᐃᔅᐸᔪᔪᑫᓐ᙮ ᓇᒧᐃ ᐅᐦᒋ ᓂᑐᐧᐁᔪᐦᑕᒧᒡ ᐊᓂᔮ ᒉᒌ ᐃᔅᐸᔪᔪᒡ᙮ ᐁᒄ ᑳ ᐄᑖᑲᓅᑦ ᐁᑎᑑ ᒋᐹ ᒥᐧᔫᔮ ᑌᔪᑯᒡ ᐊᓂᑕ ᒪᓯᓇᐦᐄᒉᐅᑲᒥᑯᐦᒡ ᒉᒌ ᐋᐸᑎᓯᑦ᙮

« Mon garçon, tu es mort. Cette machine a sonné le bip continu. Je t'ai un peu giflé et je t'ai crié de revenir. Et c'est une bonne chose que tu l'aies fait, sinon j'aurais été assez fâchée contre toi ».

Cette chambre d'hôtel, elle avait été réelle, mais elle ne l'était pas dans ce monde.

Après que Jack ait terminé toutes les séances de physiothérapie et de récupération qu'il était censé faire, il se prépara à reprendre le travail. Toutefois, juste à ce moment-là, son patron l'appela chez lui. L'entreprise ne voulait pas vraiment que Jack retourne au travail en tant qu'agent de conservation sur le terrain, déclara son patron. Avec sa nouvelle prothèse, il était capable de faire le travail, ils pouvaient le voir, et il avait toujours été un bon travailleur. Cependant, ils avaient peur d'être poursuivis en justice si quelque chose se passait mal pour Jack et sa jambe artificielle dans la forêt. Ils ne voulaient pas être tenus pour responsables. Au lieu de cela, il y avait un travail de bureau qui l'attendait et qu'ils pensaient être parfait pour lui.

"Boy, you died. That machine went into a flatline. I slapped you around a bit and yelled at you to come back. And it's a good thing you did, or I woulda been so mad at you."

That hotel room, it had been real, but it hadn't been in this world.

After Jack had finished all of the physiotherapy and recuperation stuff he was supposed to do, he got ready to head back to work. But just then, his boss called him at home. The company didn't actually want Jack back at work as a conservation officer in the field, his boss said. With his new prosthesis, he was able to do the work, they could see that, and he had always been a good worker. But they were afraid of being sued if something went wrong for Jack and his artificial leg in the bush. They didn't want the liability. Instead, there was a desk job waiting that they thought would be perfect for him.

ᓂᒧᐃ ᐅᐦᒋ ᐧᐄᐦ ᐋᐱᑎᓰᐤ ᒑᒃ ᐊᓂᑖᐦ ᐲᐦᑎᑭᒥᐦᒡ ᒥᓯᓂᐦᐄᒑᐅᑭᒥᑯᐦᒡ᙮ ᐋᑯᑖᐦ ᑳ ᐄᔑ ᐧᐃᔮᔨᐦᑎᐦᒃ᙮

ᒥᒄ ᒫᒃ ᒑᒃ ᓂᒧᐃ ᐅᐦᒋ ᐧᐄᐦ ᐴᓃᐤ ᐋᐦ ᐄᐦᑐᑎᐦᒃ ᒑᐧᑳᔨᐤ᙮ ᑭᔮᐦ ᒥᔥᑏᐦ ᒌᐦ ᒋᔅᑯᑎᒫᓲ᙮ ᒌᐦ ᒋᔅᑯᑎᒫᓲ ᐄᔨᔨᐅᐃᔨᐦᑎᐧᐃᓂᔨᐤ ᐊᓂᑖᐦ ᓂᑑᐦᐆᔅᒌᐦᒡ, ᑭᔮᐦ ᒌᐦ ᒋᔅᑯᑎᒫᓲ ᐋᐦ ᓈᓈᑭᒋᐦᑖᑭᓂᐧᐃᐧᐃᔨᒡ ᐊᔅᒌᔨᐤ ᑭᔮᐦ ᓂᑐᐦᐅᐧᐃᓂᔨᐤ ᑭᔮᐦ ᐋᐦ ᓅᒋᔥᑯᑎᐧᐋᓂᐧᐃᐧᐃᔨᒡ᙮ ᓂᔥᑐ ᐊᔨᒧᐧᐃᓐᐦ ᒌᐦ ᒋᔅᒑᔨᐦᑎᒻ᙮ ᒌᐦ ᐃᐦᑎᑯᓂᔨᐤ ᒦᓐ ᑯᑎᒋᔨᐤ ᒑᐧᑳᔨᐤ ᒐ ᒌᐦ ᐃᐦᑐᑎᐦᒃ᙮

ᐊᓂᔮᐦ ᒫᒃ ᑳ ᐧᐃᓂᐦᑖᑦ ᐅᔅᑳᑦ ᑭᔮᐦ ᐅᑖᐱᑎᓲᐧᐃᓐ ᓂᒧᐃ ᐅᐦᒋ ᐧᐋᐦᑎᓂᔨᐤ᙮ ᐋᑯᑎᐦ ᑳ ᐱᒋᔅᑖᔨᒧᑦ, ᐃᔮᒄ ᑳ ᐃᐦᑎᐦᒃ ᑳ ᐄᔥᐱᔑ ᐱᒫᑎᓰᑦ, ᐋᐦ ᒋᔅᑎᒫᒑᔨᒦᓯᑦ᙮ ᒥᔥᑏᐦ ᒌᐦ ᒥᓂᐦᐧᑳᐤ ᑭᔮᐦ ᓂᒧᐃ ᒑᐧᑳᔨᐤ ᐅᐦᒋ ᐃᐦᑐᑎᒻ = ᐋᑯᑎᐦ ᐊᑎᑎᐤ ᒦᓐ ᓈᔥᒡ ᑳ ᒫᑯᐦᐄᑯᑦ ᐋᐦ ᔖᑳᐅᐱᔨᑦ ᑭᔮᐦ ᒎᔥ ᓂᑐᐦᑯᔨᓂᑭᒥᑯᐦᒡ ᐋᐦ ᐄᐦᑖᑦ, ᑭᔮᐦ ᒌᐦ ᑯᐧᑲᑖᔨᐦᑎᒻ ᒐ ᐃᔮᔪᐧᐃᐦᐄᓯᑦ ᑭᔮᐦ ᒥᔥᑏᐦ ᒌᐦ ᐅᑎᓂᒻ ᓂᑐᐦᑯᔨᓐᐦ᙮ ᓂᒧᐃ ᑭᔨᐧᐹ ᑖᐧᐹ ᒋᔥᒋᐧᐋ ᐅᐦᒋ ᐧᐄᐦ ᐃᔮᔪᐧᐃᐦᐄᓲ, ᒥᒄ ᒫᒃ ᓈᔥᒡ ᐄᔨᐦᒡ ᐋᐦ ᒌᐦ ᐄᔑᓈᑯᓂᔨᒡ ᐅᐱᒫᑎᓲᐧᐃᓐ ᐊᓂᔮ ᑳ ᐄᔑ ᐅᐧᐃᔮᔨᐦᑎᐦᒃ ᑭᔮᐦ ᑳ ᐄᔑ ᐹᐧᔖᔨᐦᑎᐦᒃ ᒑ ᐄᔑᓈᑯᓂᔨᒡ᙮ ᓈᔥᒡ ᐋᐦ ᒌᐦ ᐅᐧᐋᓈᔨᐦᑎᐦᒃ᙮ ᒌᐦ ᓂᑎᐧᐋᔨᐦᑎᒻ ᒦᓐ ᒑ ᒥᔪᐱᒫᑎᓲᑦ᙮ ᒌᐦ ᓂᑎᐧᐋᔨᐦᑎᒻ ᒑ ᒥᐧᔮᔨᒧᑦ ᑭᔮᐦ ᒑ ᐃᔮᐱᑖᔨᒫᑭᓂᐧᐃᑦ᙮ ᒌᐦ ᓂᑎᐧᐋᔨᒫᐤ ᐊᐧᐋᔨᐤᐦ ᒑ ᐄᑎᑯᑦ ᒥᓯᐧᐋ ᒑᐧᑳᔨᐤ ᒑ ᒥᔪᐱᔨᔨᒡ᙮ ᑭᔮᐦ ᑭᐱᐦ ᒌᐦ ᒥᔮᔨᐦᑎᒻ ᒌ ᐄᑎᑯᑦ

ᓇᒧᐃ ᒫᒃ ᒦᒋᓲᓈᐦᑎᑯᐦᒡ ᐅᐦᒋ ᐧᐄ ᐊᐴ ᐁ ᐋᐸᑎᓯᑦ᙮ ᐁᑯᓐ ᒫᒃ ᑳ ᐃᔑᓈᑯᓂᔨᒡ, ᓇᒧᐃ ᒦᓐ ᐅᐦᒋ ᐋᐸᑎᓲ ᐊᓂᑌ᙮

ᒎᔥ ᒌ ᐃᔑᓈᑯᓲ ᒑᒃ ᐊᓐ ᐊᐧᐁᓐ ᑳ ᑫᔥᑎᓈᑌᔨᐦᑕᐦᒃ ᑫ ᒥᔫᐸᔨᔨᒡ ᑫᐧᑳᔫ᙮ ᒥᔅᑕᐦᐄ ᒌ ᒋᔅᑫᔨᐦᑕᒻ ᑫᐧᑳᔫ ᒋᔅᑯᑕᒫᑫᐅᑲᒥᑯᐦᒡ ᐁᒌ ᒋᔅᑯᑕᒫᓱᑦ᙮ ᒌ ᒋᔅᑯᑕᒫᓲ ᑲᔪ ᐄᓅ ᐃᐦᑐᐧᐃᓂᔫ ᓅᐦᒋᒦᐦᒡ ᐁ ᐃᐦᑖᓅᔨᒡ, ᑲᔪ ᒌ ᒋᔅᑯᑕᒫᓲ ᐊᓂᔫ ᑳ ᐄᑖᐸᑎᓯᑦ ᐊᐧᐁᓲᔅ ᑲᔪ ᐊᔅᒋᔫ ᓀᔅᑕ ᐁ ᓅᑕᑫᔅᓅᔨᒡ ᐁ ᓇᓈᑲᒋᐦᑖᑲᓅᔨᒡ, ᑲᔪ ᐋᔥᑕᐧᐁᐦᐄᑫᔫ ᒌᔑ ᒋᔅᑯᑕᒫᓲ᙮ ᓂᔥᑐᔨᒡ ᒌᔑ ᑲᔅᒋᐦᐆ ᐁ ᐃᔑ ᐊᔨᒥᑦ᙮ ᐧᐄᐸᒡ ᒋᐹᐦᒌ ᒥᔅᑰ ᐋᐸᑎᓲ᙮

ᒥᒄ ᒫᒃ ᐊᓂᔫ ᐁᒌ ᒋᒥᔑᑲᓅᔨᒡ ᐅᔅᑳᑦ ᐁᒄ ᒫᒃ ᐁᒌ ᒪᓈᑲᓅᑦ ᐊᓂᑌ ᑳ ᐋᐸᑎᓯᑦ ᐁᑯᑦ ᑳᐧᐄ ᐋᔨᒣᔨᐦᑕᐦᒃ ᐁᑳ ᐅᐦᒋ ᔮᐧᐋᐸᐦᑕᒨᒪᑲᓂᔨᐧᑳᐤ ᐊᓂᔫ ᓃᔕᔨᒡ ᐁᒌ ᐃᔅᐸᔨᑦ᙮ ᐁᑯᑦ ᑳ ᐋᔨᒣᔨᐦᑕᐦᒃ, ᐁᒄ ᔮᒄ ᑳ ᐃᑕᒪᐦᒋᐦᐅᑦ ᒨᔮᒻ ᓈᔅᒡ ᐁ ᒋᔅᑎᒫᑎᓲᑦ ᐁᒌ ᐃᑌᔨᒥᓱᑦ᙮ ᐁᒄ ᑳ ᒥᓂᐦᐧᑫᑦ ᒥᔅᑕᐦᐄ ᐁ ᒥᓂᐦᐧᑫᑦ ᑲᔪ ᓇᒧᐃ ᒥᒍᓐ ᐅᐦᒋ ᐃᐦᑑᑕᒻ ᑫᐧᑳᔫ ᐱᔑᒄ ᒥᒄ ᐁ ᐊᔭᐱᑦ = ᐅᔫ ᒫᒃ ᐁᒌ ᐃᐦᑎᑦ ᐁᑎᑑ ᒌ ᐊᑎ ᔒᐧᐋᑲᒥᐦᐧᑫᐸᔫᐤ ᑲᔪ ᒌ ᐋᐦᐧᑫᔨᐦᑕᒻ ᐋᔅᑰ ᐋᐦᑯᓰᐅᑲᒥᑯᐦᒡ ᐁᒌ ᑲᓇᐧᐁᔨᒫᑲᓅᑦ᙮ ᑫᒃ ᒌ ᐅᑎᐦᒋᐸᔨᓂᔫ ᐁ ᐃᑌᔨᐦᑕᐦᒃ ᑫᒌ ᐧᐊᓈᒋᐦᐄᓱᑦ ᐁᒄ ᑳ ᐊᑯᐦᒋᐸᔨᐦᑖᑦ ᒥᐦᑫᑐ ᓂᑐᐦᑯᐃᓐᐦ᙮ ᓇᒧᐃ ᑮᐹ ᐅᐦᒋᐧᐄ ᓂᐴ ᒥᒄ ᓇᒧᐃ ᐅᐦᒋ ᒥᔪᔨᐦᑕᒻ ᐊᓂᔫ ᐁ ᐃᔅᐸᔨᑦ ᐁᑳ ᐅᐦᒋ ᐯᔓᐧᐁᔨᐦᑕᒃ ᑫ ᐃᔅᐸᔨᑦ᙮ ᒌᐧᐄ ᐧᐊᐧᐋᓀᔨᐦᑕᒻ ᑖᓐ ᑫᒌ ᐃᐦᑎᑦ᙮ ᒌ ᐳᑯᓭᔨᒨ ᑌᑲᔥ ᑫᒌ ᒦᓂᐧᐋᑎᓰᑦ᙮ ᒌᐧᐄ ᒥᔪᔨᒨ ᑲᔪ ᒌ ᓂᑐᐧᐁᔨᑫᐤ

Jack ne voulait pas travailler dans un bureau. Ça réglait la question pour lui.

Jusqu'à présent, Jack avait été une personne de type optimiste. Et il avait une bonne éducation. Il avait étudié les méthodes traditionnelles des Cris sur le territoire, il avait étudié pour devenir garde-chasse, agent de conservation de la faune et pompier. Il pouvait parler trois langues. Il avait des options.

Toutefois, perdre une jambe et un emploi dans l'intervalle de quelques semaines, c'était un peu trop. Il abandonna son optimisme et, pour la première fois de sa vie, il commença à s'apitoyer sur son sort. Il se mit à boire et à rester assis à profusion, ce qui a entraîna une augmentation de ses comas diabétiques et hypoglycémiques, et de ses séjours à l'hôpital. Il pensa même à se suicider et avala un flacon de pilules. Il ne voulait pas vraiment mourir, mais sa vie se déroulait si différemment de ce qu'il avait prévu et de ce à quoi il s'était attendu. C'était déroutant. Il voulait que toute cette maladie cesse. Il voulait du réconfort et de l'attention. Il voulait que quelqu'un lui dise que tout irait bien. Et ce serait

Jack didn't want to work at a desk. That was the end of that.

So far Jack had been an optimistic sort of guy. And he had quite a bit of education. He had studied traditional Cree ways on the land, he had studied to be a game warden and a wildlife conservation officer and a firefighter. He could speak three languages. He had options.

But losing a leg and a job in a matter of weeks was a bit much. He let go of his optimism and, for the first time in his life, he began to feel really sorry for himself. He did a whole lot of drinking and a whole lot of sitting around – which led to more diabetic and hypoglycemic comas and hospital stays. He even thought about killing himself and swallowed a bottle of pills. He didn't actually want to die, but his life was turning out so differently from what he had planned and expected. It was confusing. He wanted all this sickness to stop. He wanted comfort and attention. He wanted someone to tell him it would be all right. And it'd sure be nice to have someone tell him what a guy like him was supposed to do now,

ᐊᐧᐋᔨᐤᐦ ᑖᓂᑖᐦ ᒑ ᒌᐦ ᐃᐦᑎᒃ, ᔖᔥ ᐋᑳ ᐅᔅᑳᑎᒃ ᑭᔮᐦ ᐋᐦ ᒌᐦ ᐧᐃᓂᐦᑖᑦ ᐅᑖᐱᑎᓲᐧᐃᓐ᙮

ᒥᒄ ᒫᒃ ᓂᒧᐃ ᐅᐦᒋ ᐃᐦᑖᔨᐤᐦ ᐊᐧᐋᔨᐤᐦ ᒑ ᒌᐦ ᐧᐄᐦᑎᒫᑯᑦ ᐊᓂᔮ ᒑ ᒌᐦ ᐃᐦᑎᒃ ᑭᔮᐦ ᒫᒃ ᒑ ᒌᐦ ᐋᐦᒋᐱᔨᐦᑖᑦ ᐊᓂᔮ ᐋᑎ ᐃᔨᔅᐱᔨᑦ᙮ ᐊᓂᑎᐦ ᒫᒃ ᒑ ᐄᔥᐱᒋ ᐃᐦᑖᑦ ᐊᓂᑎᐦ ᓈᔥᒡ ᐋᑳ ᒥᐧᔮᔨᐦᑎᐦᒃ, ᑭᔮᐦ ᐋᑳ ᓈᔥᑎᔨᐤ ᒑᐧᑳᔨᐤ ᐃᐦᑐᑎᐦᑳ ᒥᒄ ᐋᐦ ᒥᓂᐦᐧᑳᑦ ᐋᐦ ᐄᑖᐱᑎᓲᑦ ᑭᔮᐦ ᐋᑳ ᓈᔥᑎᔨᐤ ᒑᐧᑳᔨᐤ ᐃᐦᑐᑎᐦᒃ, ᐋᑯᑎᐦ ᐊᓂᑎᐦ ᒨᔥ ᒑ ᐃᐦᑖᑦ ᐊᓂᑎᐦ ᐋᑳ ᒥᐧᔮᔨᐦᑎᐦᒃ᙮ ᐊᔮᐧᐋᐤ ᐋᐦ ᐅᔅᒋᐱᒫᑎᓯᔨᐤᐦ ᐅᔅᑯᓯᔅᐦ᙮ ᓂᒧᐃ ᐅᐦᒋ ᓂᑎᐧᐋᔨᒫᐤ ᐊᓂᔮᐦ ᐅᑎᐧᐋᔑᔒᒻᐦ ᒑᐦ ᒌᐦ ᐄᑖᔨᐦᑎᒥᑯᑦ ᓈᔥᑎᔨᐤ ᒋᔥᒋᐧᐋ ᐋᐦ ᒌᐦ ᐱᒋᔅᒑᔨᒧᑦ᙮

ᐧᐄᔨ ᒥᒄ ᒋᑭ ᒌᐦ ᐄᔑᓈᑯᓂᔨᐤ ᒑ ᒌᐦ ᐋᐦᒋᔥᑖᑦ ᒑᐧᑳᔨᐤ ᐄᔨᐦᐤ ᒑ ᒌᐦ ᐄᔑᓈᑯᓂᔨᒡ ᐅᐱᒫᑎᓲᐧᐃᓐ᙮

ᓂᒧᐃ ᓈᔥᒡ ᐅᐦᒋ ᐧᐄᐦ ᐃᔮᐦᑖᔨᐦᑎᒻ ᓃᔥᑎᒻ, ᒑᒃ ᑳ ᒫᒥᑐᓈᔨᐦᑎᐦᒃ ᑖᓂᑖᐦ ᒑ ᒌᐦ ᐃᐦᑎᒃ ᒦᓐ ᑳᐤ ᐧᐄᔨ ᒑ ᒌᐦ ᐱᒥᓃᓯᑦ᙮ ᒨᔥ ᒌᐦ ᐄᑖᔨᐦᑎᒻ ᒑ ᐧᐄᒋᐦᐋᑦ ᑭᔮᐦ ᒑ ᐋᐱᑎᔒᔥᑎᐧᐋᑦ ᐊᐧᐋᔑᔥᐦ᙮ ᒌᐦ ᒋᔅᑯᑎᒫᓲ ᐊᓂᑎᐦ ᒑ ᒌᐦ ᐅᐦᒋ ᒋᐱᒋᐦᐋᑭᓂᐧᐃᐧᐃᔨᐤᐦ ᐋᐦ ᐄᑖᔨᐦᑎᒥᔨᐤᐦ ᐊᐧᐋᔨᐤᐦ ᐋᐦ ᐧᐄᐦ ᐃᔮᔪᐧᐃᐦᐄᓯᔨᐤᐦ = ᐧᐄᔨ ᒫᒃ ᑭᔮᐦ ᐋᐦ ᒌᐦ ᐅᑎᓂᐦᒃ ᓂᑐᐦᑯᔨᓐᐦ ᐊᓂᔮ ᐋᐦ ᐧᐄᐦ ᐃᐦᑐᑖᓯᑦ = ᒌᐦ ᒋᔅᒑᔨᒫᐤ ᑭᔮᐦ ᐄᔨᔨᐤ ᐊᐧᐋᔑᔥᐦ ᓈᔥᒡ ᐋᑳ ᒥᔪᐱᔨᔨᐤᐦ᙮ ᐧᑳᐧᔖᓐ

ᐊᐧᐁᔫ ᒉᒌ ᒥᔫᐦᑳᑯᑦ᙮ ᒌᐧᐄ ᐯᐦᑕᐧᐁᐤ ᐊᐧᐁᔫ ᐁ ᐃᑎᑯᑦ ᒉ ᒥᔫᐸᔨᑦ᙮ ᒋᐹ ᒥᔫᐦᑕᒻ ᒌ ᐧᐄᐦᑕᒫᑰᑯᐸᓀ ᐊᐧᐁᔫ ᑖᓐ ᒋᐹ ᐃᐦᑑ ᐋᑦ ᐁ ᓂᐸᑌᑳᑌᐤ ᑲᔦ ᐁᑳ ᐊᔮᑦ ᐋᐸᑎᓯᐧᐃᓂᔫ᙮

ᓇᒧᐃ ᒫᒃ ᒥᑐᓐ ᐅᐦᒋ ᐃᐦᑖᔫ ᐊᐧᐁᔫ ᒉᒌ ᓈᑕᒫᑯᑦ ᒉᒌ ᐧᐄᐦᑕᒫᑯᑦ ᑖᓐ ᒋᐱᒌ ᐃᐦᑑ ᒉᒌ ᐅᐦᒋ ᐧᑫᔅᒋᐸᔨᔨᐤ ᐊᓂᔫ ᒉᐧᑳᐤ ᐁ ᐃᔑ ᓇᒋᔅᑲᐦᒃ᙮ ᒥᒋᐦᐱᓐ ᐁᑳ ᐋᐦᒌᐤ ᐃᔅᐸᔨᓂᔨᒉ ᐅᐱᒫᑎᓲᐧᐃᓐ ᐁᑳ ᒥᔦᔨᐦᑕᐦᒃ ᑲᔦ ᐱᔑᒄ ᒥᓂᐦᐧᑫᑌ ᐁᑳ ᐃᐦᑑᑕᐦᒃ ᑯᑕᒋᔫ ᒉᐧᑳᔫ ᒋᑲᒌ ᐃᔑᓈᑯᓂᔫ ᐊᓂᔫ ᒋᐦᒋᐧᐁ ᒉᒌ ᐄᑖᑎᓲᑦ᙮ ᒌ ᐃᐦᑖᔫ ᑲᔦ ᓵᔅ ᐆᑕᐧᐋᔒᒥᔥ ᐁ ᓈᐯᓯᐧᐃᔨᐤ᙮ ᓇᒧᐃ ᐅᐦᒋ ᓂᑐᐧᐁᔨᐦᑕᒻ ᒉᒌ ᐃᑌᔨᒥᑯᑦ ᑌᑭᔅ ᐁᒌ ᐴᓈᐸᐦᑕᒃ ᒉᐧᑳᔫ᙮

ᐁᒄ ᑮᐹ ᑳ ᐃᔑᓈᑯᓂᔨᒡ ᐧᐄ ᒉᐧᐄ ᒋᔅᒉᔨᐦᑕᐦᒃ ᑖᓐ ᒉ ᐃᐦᑎᑦ ᐁᐧᐄ ᐧᐄᒋᐦᐄᓯᑦ᙮

ᓃᔥᑕᒻ ᓇᒧᐃ ᐅᐦᒋ ᐧᐄ ᓵᐯᔨᐦᑕᒻ ᒉᐧᑳᔫ ᒉᒌ ᐃᐦᑑᑕᐦᒃ ᒉᒃ ᑳ ᒫᒥᑐᓀᔨᐦᑕᐦᒃ ᑖᓐ ᒋᐹᒌ ᐃᐦᑑ ᐁᐧᐄ ᐱᒫᒋᐦᐄᓯᑦ᙮ ᐊᓂᑌ ᐅᑖᐦᒡ ᒨᔥ ᒌ ᐃᑌᔨᐦᑕᒻ ᒉᒌ ᐧᐄᒋᐦᐋᑦ ᐅᔅᒋᓃᒎᐦ᙮ ᒌ ᒋᔅᒉᔨᒣᐤ ᑖᓐ ᐁ ᐃᔅᐸᔨᔨᐤ ᐅᐱᒫᑎᓲᐧᐃᓂᔨᐦᐤ᙮ ᓵᔅ ᐊᓂᑌ ᐯᒋ ᒌ ᒋᔅᑯᑕᒫᓲ ᑖᓐ ᒋᐹ ᐃᐦᑎᓈᓅ ᐁᐧᐄ ᒋᐱᐦᒋᐦᐋᑲᓅᑦ ᐊᐧᐁᓐ ᑳ ᐧᑫᑌᔨᐦᑕᐦᒃ ᒉᒌ ᐃᔅᐧᑳᓇᐦᒃ ᐅᐱᒪᑎᓲᐧᐃᓐ = ᐁᐅᒄ ᐆ ᓈᐯᐤ ᑳᐧᐄ ᓂᐱᐦᐄᓯᑦ ᐯᔭᒄ ᐴᑕᐃ ᓂᑐᐦᑯᐄᓐᐦ ᐁᒌ ᐊᑯᐦᒋᐸᔨᐦᑖᑦ᙮ ᒌ ᒋᔅᒉᔨᐦᑕᒻ ᐁ ᐃᐦᑖᔨᐤ ᐅᔅᒋᓃᒎᐦ ᒥᔅᑕᐦᐄ ᐁ ᐃᔑ

certainement bien que quelqu'un lui dise ce qu'un type comme lui était censé faire désormais, avec une jambe et un travail en moins.

missing a leg and a job.

Le problème était qu'il n'y *avait* personne, vraiment, qui pouvait lui dire ce qu'il devait faire ou qui pouvait changer sa situation. Tant qu'il était dans une situation qu'il n'aimait pas et tant qu'il ne faisait rien d'autre pour y remédier que de boire et demeurer assis, il continuerait à être dans la situation qu'il n'aimait pas. Il avait aussi un nouveau fils désormais. Il ne voulait pas que son enfant pense que son père avait abandonné.

The problem was that there *was* no one, really, who could tell him what to do or who could change his situation. As long as he was in a situation he didn't like, and as long as he did nothing about it but drink and sit around, he would continue to be in the situation he didn't like. He had a new son now too. He didn't want his kid to think that his dad had given up.

Il devrait résoudre sa situation par lui-même.

He would have to figure it out for himself.

À contrecœur, dans les premiers temps, Jack se ressaisit et commença à réfléchir à d'autres moyens de gagner sa vie. Il avait toujours voulu travailler avec des enfants. Il les comprenait. Il avait suivi un cours de prévention du suicide – marrant pour un type qui avait avalé un flacon de pilules – et il savait que certains enfants cris avaient des problèmes. Il avait peut-être quelque chose à offrir.

Begrudgingly at first, Jack pulled himself together and started to think about other ways he could make a living. He had always wanted to work with kids. He understood them. He had taken a course in suicide prevention – funny for a guy who had swallowed a bottle of pills – and he knew some Cree kids were in trouble. Maybe he had something to offer.

ᐃᐦᑎᑯᓂᔨᒋᒑ ᐊᓂᑖᐦ ᒑ ᒌᐦ ᐄᔑ ᐧᐄᒋᐦᑖᑦ ᐆᔮ᙮

ᒥᑯ ᒫᒃ ᐊᓂᔮ ᐅᔅᑳᑦ, ᐊᓂᔮ ᐅᔅᑳᑦ ᑳ ᒫᔮᑎᓂᔨᒡ ᑮᔮᐦ ᑳ ᒥᓂᔑᑭᓂᐧᐃᐧᐃᔨᒡ, ᓈᔥᒡ ᐋᑳ ᐅᐦᒋ ᒥᐧᔮᔨᐦᑎᐦᒃ ᐊᓂᔮ ᒥᔅᑳᑎᐦᑳᓂᔨᐤ ᑳ ᒥᔮᑭᓂᐧᐃᑦ ᑳ ᐄᔅᐱᔨᐦᐄᑯᑦ ᐋᑳ ᒥᔫᔥᑭᐦᒃ ᑮᔮᐦ ᐋᐦ ᐋᐦᑯᐦᐄᑯᑦ ᑮᔮᐦ ᐋᐦ ᒥᓂᐱᔨᔨᒡᐦ ᐅᔑᑮᐦ ᐅᐦᒋ ᐊᓂᔮ ᐋᑳ ᒥᔫᔥᑭᐦᒃ, ᑮᔮᐦ ᑳ ᐋᑎ ᒫᔮᑎᓂᔨᒡ, ᐊᓂᑖᐦ ᐧᒫᓐᑎᓈᐧᔮᑦ ᑳ ᐄᑎᔑᐦᐧᐋᑭᓂᐧᐃᑦ ᒑ ᒌᐦ ᐧᐄᒋᐦᐋᑭᓂᐧᐃᑦ ᔖᔥ ᑭᔨᐧᐹ ᐋᐦ ᐃᔨᑮᔮᔮᐦᑎᐦᒃ ᐊᓂᔮ ᒑ ᐃᐦᑐᑎᐧᐋᑭᓂᐧᐃᑦ ᐆᔮ ᐋᐦ ᐧᐄᐦ ᐄᔑ ᐧᐄᒋᐦᐋᑭᓂᐧᐃᑦ᙮

ᓈᐦᐋᐤ ᒫᒃ ᒦᓐ ᑳ ᐄᔅᐱᔨᔨᒡ = ᒑᒃ ᓂᑐᐦᑯᔨᓂᑭᒥᑯᐦᒡ ᒌᐦ ᐃᐦᑖᐤ ᐋᐦ ᐧᐄ ᐧᐄᒋᐦᑖᑭᓂᐧᐃᐧᐃᔨᒡ ᐊᓂᑎᐦ ᑳ ᒥᓂᔑᑭᓂᐧᐃᐧᐃᔨᒡ ᐅᔅᑳᑦ, ᒦᓐ ᑳ ᐃᐦᑐᑎᑭᓂᐧᐃᐧᐃᔨᒡ ᐋᐦ ᐧᐄᐦ ᑯᔨᐧᑳᔑᑭᐧᐃᐦᑖᑭᓂᐧᐃᐧᐃᔨᒡ ᐊᓂᔮ ᐋᐦ ᒫᔮᑎᓂᔨᒡ ᐊᓂᑖᐦ ᐅᐦᒋ ᐅᔅᑳᑎᐦᒡ, ᑮᔮᐦ ᑳ ᐃᐦᑐᑎᑭᓂᐧᐃᐧᐃᔨᒡ ᐋᐦ ᒋᔥᑖᐹᐅᑖᑭᓂᐧᐃᐧᐃᔨᒡ ᑮᔮᐦ ᓂᑐᐦᑯᔨᓂᔨᐤ ᐋᐦ ᐱᒋᔅᑎᓂᑭᓂᐧᐃᐧᐃᔨᒡ, ᓂᒧᐃ ᒫᒃ ᐅᐦᒋ ᐧᐄᒋᐦᐄᑰ ᑮᔮᐦ ᑳ ᐋᑎ ᒫᐦᒋᐱᔨᔨᒡᐦ ᐊᓂᔮᐦ ᐅᔑᑮᐦ, ᐋᑯᐦ ᒦᓐ ᑳ ᑭᓂᐧᐋᐱᐦᑎᒥᔨᒡᐦ ᓂᑐᐦᑯᔨᓐᐦ᙮ ᑳ ᐄᑖᑭᓂᐧᐃᑦ ᒦᓐ ᒑ ᒫᒋᔑᑭᓂᐧᐃᐧᐃᔨᒡ᙮ ᐋᔫᐧᐃᑯ ᐊᓂᔮ ᐋᔮᐱᒡ ᒦᓐ ᐅᔅᑳᑦ, ᐊᓂᑖᐦ ᐊᑎᑎᐤ ᐄᔥᐲᒥᐦᒡ, ᐄᔥᐱᒥᐦᒡ ᐊᓂᑎᐦ ᐅᐦᒋᑯᓂᐦᒡ᙮ ᒦᓐ᙮

ᓇᒋᔥᑲᒥᔨᒡ ᐅᐱᒫᑎᓰᐧᐃᓂᔨᐦᒡ ᐁ ᐋᔨᒥᐦᐄᑯᔨᒡ᙮ ᐃᐦᑕᑯᓂᔨᒉ ᑖᓐ ᓂᐱᐦᒌ ᐃᔑ ᐧᐋᐧᐄᒋᐦᐋᐅᒡ, ᒌ ᐃᑌᔨᐦᑕᒻ᙮

ᐁᑯ ᒦᓐ ᑳ ᐃᐦᑕᑯᓂᔨᒡ ᐁ ᐃᔅᐸᔨᑦ = ᐋᐦᑯᔩᐅᑲᒥᑯᐦᒡ ᒌ ᐃᐦᑖᐤ ᐁᒌ ᒥᔫᓂᔨᒡ ᐊᓂᔫ ᐅᔅᑳᒡ ᐊᓂᑕ ᑳ ᒋᒥᔑᑲᓄᔨᒡ, ᐁᑯ ᑮᐹ ᒦᓐ ᑳ ᐅᑕᐦᐄᑲᓄᔨᒡ ᐊᓂᔫ ᒥᐳ ᑳ ᒋᔅᑖᐳᑖᑲᓄᔨᒡ ᑲᔦ ᓂᑐᐦᑯᐃᓂᔫ ᒌ ᐊᔥᑖᑲᓅᔫ ᐊᓂᑕ, ᐋᑦ ᒫᒃ ᐅᔫ ᐁᒌ ᐃᐦᑑᑕᐧᐋᑲᓅᑦ ᓇᒧᐃ ᔮᐸᒡ ᐅᐦᒌ ᒥᐧᔮᔫ ᐅᔅᑳᑦ ᐁᑯ ᒦᓐ ᑳ ᑲᓇᐧᐋᐸᐦᑕᒥᔨᔨᒡ ᓂᑐᐦᑯᐃᓐᐦ᙮ ᑳ ᐄᑖᑲᓅᑦ ᒦᓐ ᒉ ᒫᒋᔑᑲᓄᔨᒡ ᐊᓂᔫ ᐅᔅᑳᑦ, ᐃᔅᐱᒦᔔᔥ ᐊᓂᑕ ᐊᓂᔫ ᐅᐦᒋᑯᓐ᙮ ᐁᐧᑫᔅᐦ, ᒦᓐ ᒋᑲ ᒦᒋᔔᑲᓄᔫ᙮

Mais cette jambe, la mauvaise jambe qui avait déjà été amputée, le gênait à nouveau. La prothèse frottait fortement sur le moignon. Parfois, elle frottait jusqu'au sang, puis la blessure s'infectait et il devait aller à Montréal pour le contrôle des infections; tout cela lui était si familier.

But that leg, the bad leg that had already been amputated, was bothering him again. The prosthesis rubbed badly against the stump. Sometimes the skin rubbed right off and then it got infected and he would have to go to Montréal for infection control and it was all so familiar.

Jack était à l'hôpital pour être soigné d'une infection du moignon, et, bien sûr, ils posèrent des drains pour évacuer les fluides de la chair, et, bien sûr, ils nettoyèrent la zone avec des produits antibiotiques et appliquèrent des traitements et, bien sûr, les traitements ne fonctionnaient pas et la chair était rongée et, bien sûr, le médecin y jeta un coup d'œil. Il dit qu'ils allaient devoir amputer. La même jambe, plus haut, au-dessus du genou. À nouveau.

Wouldn't you know – Jack was in the hospital being treated for infection in the stump, and again they had the drains carrying fluid out of the flesh, and again they were washing the area with antibiotics and applying treatments, and again the treatments weren't working and the flesh was being eaten away, and again the doctor took a look. And said they were going to have to amputate. The same leg, up higher, above the knee. Again.

ᒥᑯ ᐄᔑ ᐑᐦᐧᑳᐤ ᒑᒃ ᐋᐦ ᐄᔨᔨᐅᔨᒥᑦ᙮ ᒌᐦ ᐑᐦ ᐑᐦᐧᑳᐤ ᐋᐦ ᐚᒥᔥᑎᑯᔒᐅᔨᒥᑦ ᑮᔮᐦ ᐋᐦ ᐱᔥᑎᐧᑳᔮᐅᔨᒥᑦ, ᒥᑯ ᓂᒥ ᐅᐦᒋ ᐑᐦ ᒋᔅᒑᔨᐦᑎᔮᐤ ᐊᓂᔮ ᓂᑐᐦᑯᔨᓐᐦ ᑮᔮᐦ ᓂᑐᐦᑯᔨᓂᔅᐧᑳᐤᐦ ᐋᐦ ᐑᐦᐧᑳᑦ᙮ ᒥᑯ ᒦᓐ ᑳ ᐚᐑᐦᐧᑳᑦ ᐋᐦ ᐄᔨᔨᐅᔨᒥᑦ ᑮᔮᐦ ᒌᐦ ᐹᐦᑎᒥᔨᒋᒑᓂᐦᐄ ᐊᓂᔮᐦ ᐊᓂᑎᐦ ᑳ ᐃᐦᑖᔨᒡᐦ ᐊᔨᒧᐎᓂᔨᐤ ᐋᑳ ᓂᐦᑖ ᐅᐦᒋ ᐹᐦᑎᒥᔨᒡᐦ᙮

ᓂᒧᐃ ᓈᔥᒡ ᒥᐦᒑᑐᒌᔑᐧᑳᐤᐦ, ᑳ ᐄᔅᐱᑖᑭᓂᐎᑦ ᐊᓂᑖᐦ ᒑ ᒫᒋᐧᔖᑭᓂᐎᑦ ᑮᔮᐦ ᑳ ᑯᔥᑯᐱᔨᑦ᙮ ᐊᓂᑎᐦ ᐋᐱᐦᑎᐤ ᐅᐧᐹᒥᐦᒡ ᐋᑯᑎᐦ ᑳᐦ ᒋᒥᔑᑭᓂᐎᐎᔨᑯᐱᓈ ᐊᓂᔮ ᐅᔅᑳᑦ᙮

ᐊᓂᔮ ᒫᒃ ᒫᐦᒋᒡ ᑳ ᒋᓯᐚᓯᑦ ᑮᔮᐦ ᑳ ᒋᔅᑎᒫᒑᔨᒦᓯᑦ ᒑᒃ ᓂᒧᐃ ᓈᔥᑎᔨᓯ ᐅᐦᒋ ᐑᒋᐦᐄᑯᐦ᙮ ᓂᒧᐃ ᒦᓐ ᐅᐦᒋ ᐑᐦ ᐃᐦᑐᑎᒻ ᐊᓂᔮ, ᒥᑯ ᒌᐦ ᐄᑖᔨᐦᑎᒻ ᒫ ᐑᐦ ᐑᒋᐦᐄᓯᑦ᙮ ᓂᒥᔮᔨᐤ ᑳ ᓂᑎᐚᔨᐦᑎᐦᒃ ᐊᓂᔮ ᓃᔥᑎᒻ ᑳ ᐄᔑᓈᑯᓂᔨᒡ ᒥᔅᑳᑎᐦᑳᓂᔨᐤ ᑳ ᒥᔮᑭᓂᐎᑦ ᐊᓂᑖᐦ ᐅᐦᒋ ᐄᔨᔨᐤ ᓂᑐᐦᑯᔨᓈᐱᑎᓰᐎᓂᐦᒡ, ᔖᔥ ᒌᐦ ᒋᔅᒑᔨᐦᑎᒻ ᐊᓂᔮ ᑳ ᐄᔥᐱᔥ ᐋᑳ ᐅᐦᒋ ᒥᔪᐱᔨᐦᐄᑯᑦ᙮ ᐚᓵ ᒌᐦ ᐚᐦᒋᐱᔨᔨᐤ ᒦᓐ ᒫ ᒌᐦ ᒫᔮᑎᓂᔨᐤ ᐊᓂᔮ ᐅᔅᑳᑦ ᑮᔮᐦ ᒌᐦ ᒋᔅᒑᔨᐦᑎᒻ ᐊᑎᑎᐤ ᐋᐦ ᐋᔨᒥᒋᔥᑖᑯᓂᔨᒡ ᒥᔅᑳᑎᐦᑳᓂᔨᐤ ᐋᐦ ᓂᑎᐚᔨᐦᑎᐦᒃ, ᐊᓂᔮ ᑯᐃᔅᑯ ᒫ ᒌᐦ ᑖᐳᒥᔨᒡ ᑮᔮᐦ ᒫ ᔮᔨᑎᒧᔨᒡ ᑮᔮᐦ ᐋᑳ ᒫ ᐹᐱᑯᐦᐅᑯᑦ ᐅᔑᑳᐦᒡ᙮ ᐊᓂᔮᐦ ᒫᒃ ᓈᑎᐚᔨᐦᑎᐦᒃ ᒥᔅᑳᑎᐦᑳᓂᔨᐤ ᒥᑖᐦᐧᑖᐤ ᒋᔖᒥᑖᐦᑐᒥᑎᓂᐚᐦᑎᐦ ᒦᓐ ᐄᔨᐚᒡ ᒋᑭ ᐄᑎᒋᔥᑖᑯᓂᔨᐤ, ᐊᑎᑎᐤ ᓈᔥᒡ ᒥᔥᒌᐦ ᑳ ᐄᑎᒋᔥᑖᑯᓂᔨᒡ ᐊᓂᔮ ᓃᔥᑎᒻ ᑳ ᒥᔮᑭᓂᐎᑦ ᐊᓂᑖᐦ ᐅᐦᒋ

ᑖᐧᐯ ᒌ ᐚᐑᐦᐧᑫᐤ ᐁ ᐄᓅᐊᔨᒥᑦ᙮ ᒌᐑ ᐧᐁᒥᔅᑎᑰᔒᐤ ᑲᔦ ᑳᑯᔅᑫᔒ ᐚᐑᐦᐧᑫᐤ ᒥᑯ ᓇᒧᐃ ᐅᐦᒋ ᓂᑐᐧᐁᔨᒣᐤ ᐊᓂᔫᐦ ᓂᑐᐦᑯᐃᓐᐦ ᑲᔦ ᓂᑐᐦᐧᑫᐃᓂᔅᐧᑫᐤ ᑫᒌ ᓂᓯᑐᐦᑖᑯᑦ ᐁ ᐚᐑᐦᐧᑫᑦ᙮ ᐁᑯ ᐁᑎᑑ ᑳ ᐚᐑᐦᐧᑫᑦ ᐁᑯ ᐸᔅᒡ ᐊᓂᑕ ᑳ ᐃᐦᑖᔨᒡ ᑳ ᓂᓯᑐᐦᑖᑯᑦ ᓇᒧᐃ ᒫᔅᑯᒡ ᐑᔅᑳᑦ ᐅᐦᒋ ᐯᐦᑕᐧᐁᐅᒡ ᐊᐧᐁᔫᐦ ᐁ ᐃᑎᐦᑖᑯᓯᔨᒡ᙮

ᓇᒧᐃ ᒫᒃ ᒥᐦᒉᑐ ᒌᔑᑳᐤᐦ ᐁᑯ ᑳ ᒫᒋᐧᔖᑲᓅᑦ ᐁᑯ ᑳ ᐯᑯᐸᔨᑦ ᐃᔅᑯᑕᒃ ᑳ ᐃᔅᐧᑳᐤ ᑑᑕᐚᑲᓅᑦ᙮ ᑫᐧᑳᓐ ᐆ ᑌᑖᐅᐧᐹᒻ ᑳ ᐃᔅᑯᑳᑌᑦ᙮

ᐅᑖᐦᒡ ᐊᓂᑌ ᓃᔥᑕᒻ ᑳ ᒋᒥᔑᑲᓄᔨᒡ ᐅᔅᑳᑦ, ᒌ ᒥᔅᑕ ᒋᔑᐚᓰ ᒫᒃ ᑲᔦ ᓈᔅᒡ ᒌᐑ ᒋᔅᑎᒫᒉᔨᒥᑯᓲᐤ ᓇᒧᐃ ᒫᒃ ᐅᐦᒋ ᐑᒋᐦᐄᑯ ᐊᓂᔫ ᑳ ᐃᐦᑎᑦ᙮ ᓇᒧᐃ ᒫᒃ ᐅᐦᒋ ᓂᑐᐧᐁᔨᐦᑕᒻ ᐅᔫ ᑫᒌ ᐃᐦᑎᑦ ᒦᓐ, ᐁᐅᑯ ᑮᐹ ᐅᔫ ᓂᔥᐧᑖᐤ ᐁᑯ ᑳ ᐃᐦᑑᑕᐚᑲᓅᑦ, ᐁᑯ ᑳ ᐃᑌᔨᐦᑕᐦᒃ ᑫᐑ ᐑᒋᐦᐄᓱᑦ᙮ ᐊᓂᔫ ᒫᒃ ᒥᔅᑳᑎᐦᑳᓂᔫ ᑳ ᒦᑯᑦ ᒥᔫᐱᒫᑎᓰᐎᓐ ᑳ ᓈᓈᑲᒋᐦᑖᔨᒡ ᓇᒧᐃ ᐅᐦᒋ ᒥᐧᔮᔫ, ᒌ ᒋᔅᑫᔨᐦᑕᒻ ᒫᒃ ᐅᔫ ᒑᒃ᙮ ᓈᔅᒡ ᐑᐸᒡ ᒫᓐ ᐁᒌ ᐳᑯᐦᐆᑯᑦ ᐊᓂᔫ ᒥᔅᑳᑎᐦᑳᓂᔫ, ᒌ ᐃᔑᓈᑯᓂᔫ ᒫᒃ ᐁ ᓂᑐᐧᐁᔨᐦᑕᐦᒃ ᐁᑯ ᐁ ᐅᔅᑳᔨᒡ ᐁᑎᑑ ᐁ ᔕᓀᔮᐅᓂᔨᒡ ᒧᔮᒻ ᐁ ᐃᒋᔥᑲᐦᒃ ᑲᔦ ᒧᔮᒻ ᑫᒌᔑ ᑖᐱᐦᑎᓂᔨᒡ ᐅᐧᐹᒥᐦᒡ ᐁᑳ ᐳᑯᐦᐆᑯᑦ᙮ ᒥᑖᐦᐧᑖᐤ ᒋᔕᒥᑖᐦᑐᒥᑎᓅ ᐁ ᐃᑕᒋᐦᑖᑯᓂᔨᒡ ᐁᐅᑯ ᐊᓂᔫ ᒋᐹ ᒥᐧᔮᔫ ᐋᔨᑦ ᓇᒧᐃ ᒫᒃ ᒥᑯ ᐅᐦᒌ ᐃᔥᐱᔥ ᒌᔒᐦᑲᒥᔪ ᒥᔫᐱᒫᑎᓰᐎᓐ ᐁ ᓇᓈᑲᒋᐦᑖᑲᓅᐦᒡ ᐅᐦᒋ᙮ ᐊᓂᔫ ᑕᐦᑯᐦᒡ ᐁ ᐃᔥᐱᔥ ᔕᓀᔮᐅᓂᔨᒡ ᐑᔮ

Jack sacra en cri. Il avait aussi vraiment envie de sacrer en anglais et en français, mais il ne voulait pas que les médecins et les infirmières sachent qu'il sacrait. Alors il sacra davantage en cri et les autres personnes présentes dans la salle entendirent des mots qu'elles n'avaient probablement jamais entendus auparavant.

Quelques jours plus tard, il eut sa chirurgie et se réveilla après.
Son moignon de jambe s'arrêtait désormais au milieu de l'os de la cuisse.

La dernière fois, Jack avait été rongé par la colère et l'auto-apitoiement, et cela n'avait pas aidé du tout. S'il ne voulait pas revivre cette bête situation une troisième fois, il allait devoir s'aider lui-même. La prothèse fournie par le Conseil cri de la santé (CCS) n'était pas la prothèse dont Jack avait besoin, il le savait désormais. Sa chair s'infectait si facilement qu'il avait besoin d'une prothèse beaucoup plus chère, qui s'ajusterait bien, pourrait être verrouillée en position et qui ne frotterait pas sur sa peau. Une prothèse qui coûterait dix mille dollars de plus que celle fournie par le CCS. Jack devrait payer la différence lui-même.

Jack swore in Cree. He really wanted to swear in English and French too, but he didn't want the doctors and nurses there to know he was swearing. So he just swore some more in Cree and the others in the room heard some words they had probably never heard before.

A few days after that, he went into surgery and woke up after. His leg stump now ended in the middle of his thigh bone.

Last time, Jack had been eaten up with anger and self-pity and it hadn't helped at all. If he didn't want to go through the whole stupid situation a third time, he was going to have to help himself. The prosthesis provided by the Cree Board of Health was not the prosthesis that Jack needed, he knew that now. His flesh infected so easily that he needed a much more expensive prosthesis, one that fit securely and could be locked into position and wouldn't rub off his skin. One that cost ten thousand dollars more than the prosthesis CBH provided. Jack would have to pay the difference himself.

ᐄᔨᔨᐤ ᓂᑐᐦᑯᔨᓈᐱᑎᓰᐧᐃᓂᐦᒡ᙮ ᐧᐄᔨ ᒑᒃ ᓂᑎᐧᐋᔨᐦᑖᑯᓂᔨᐤ ᒑ ᒌᐦ ᑎᐹᐦᒃ ᐊᓂᔮ ᒥᔥᑎᐤ ᒑ ᐄᑎᒋᔥᑖᑯᓂᔨᒡ᙮

ᐊᓂᔮ ᒫᒃ ᒥᑖᐦᐧᑖᐤ ᒋᔐᒥᑖᐦᑐᒥᑎᓂᐧᐋᐦᒌ ᓂᒧᐃ ᐅᐦᒋ ᐄᔥᐱᔥ ᐊᔮᐧᐋᐤ ᒑᒃ᙮ ᐋᑲ ᓂᑎᐧᐋᔨᐦᑎᐦᑳ ᒦᓐ ᓈᐦᐋᐤ ᒑ ᐄᔅᐱᔮᑦ ᔮᔨᑖ ᒋᑭ ᐧᐄᐦ ᐅᐦᑎᓈᐤ ᐊᓂᔮ ᐄᔥᐱᔥ, ᐋᑲ ᑭᔨᐧᐹ ᒦᓐ ᒑ ᒫᔮᑎᓂᔨᒡ ᑭᔮᐦ ᒦᓐ ᒑ ᒫᒋᐧᔐᑭᓂᐧᐃᑦ᙮ ᐊᓂᑖᐦ ᔕᐧᐃᔮᓂᑭᒥᑯᐦᒡ ᑳᐦ ᐄᑖᔅᑯᐦᐅᓯᑦ ᒑᒃ, ᑳ ᐋᐅᐦᐋᓯᑦ ᔕᐧᐃᔮᓐᐦ ᑭᔮᐦ ᑳ ᐅᑎᓂᒫᓯᑦ ᐊᓂᔮ ᑳ ᐋᔨᒥᒋᐦᑖᑯᓂᔨᒡ ᒥᔅᑳᑎᐦᑳᓂᔨᐤ᙮ ᓈᔥᒡ ᐋᐦ ᒌᐦ ᔑᔥᑭᒋᐦᐄᑯᑦ ᐊᓂᔮ ᑳ ᐄᔅᐱᔨᑦ ᒥᒄ ᒫᒃ ᐊᔮᐱᒡ ᒌᐦ ᐃᐦᑐᑎᒫᓰ ᒑᐧᑳᔨᐤ ᐄᔨᐦᒡ ᒑ ᒌᐦ ᐄᔅᐱᔮᑦ᙮ ᐃᔅᑯᑎᒃ ᒫᒃ ᑳ ᒥᔦᔥᑭᒨᔮᑭᓂᐧᐃᑦ ᐊᓂᔮ ᑳ ᐅᔥᑳᔮᐤ, ᑳ ᒌᐧᐋᐱᔮᑦ, ᑳ ᐊᐧᐋᔮᐱᑦ ᑭᔮᐦ ᑳ ᐋᔮᐧᐋᔑᑦ ᑳ ᐲᔥᒑᐅᐱᔮᔑᔮᒡ ᐋᐦ ᒥᓂᐦᐧᑳᑦ᙮

ᐊᓂᔮᐦ ᒫᒃ ᐋᐦ ᔐᑳᐅᐱᔮᑦ ᑭᔮᐦ ᓂᔮᓂᑯᑑᓐᐦ ᒥᒄ ᐋᐦ ᒌᐦ ᐄᔑ ᑭᐧᐃᐦᑯᔑᑦ ᐊᓂᔮ ᓈᔥᒡ ᐋᐦ ᐄᔅᑯᐱᔮᔮᒡ ᐅᔕᑳᒻ, ᑭᔮᐦ ᒥᐦᒑᐧᑖᐤ ᓂᑐᐦᑯᔨᓂᑭᒥᑯᐦᒡ ᐋᐦ ᒌᐦ ᐃᐦᑖᑦ, ᐊᔮᐱᒡ ᓂᒥ ᐅᐦᒋ ᐴᓂᔮᔮᐤ᙮ ᓂᔮᓂᑯᑑᓐᐦ ᒑᔥᑎᐦᐅᓯᒡ ᒑᒃ ᐄᓐᓯᓚᓐ, ᑳ ᒌ ᐄᑖᔮᐦᑎᐦᒃ ᐋᐅᒄ ᑳᑭᔮᐦ ᐧᐋᐦᒋ ᐃᐦᑎᔮᓐ ᐋᐦ ᒥᓂᐦᐧᑳᔮᓐ, ᐅᔮ ᒫᒃ ᐋᔑᓈᑯᓂᔮᐧᑲ, ᐊᓂᔮᐦ ᓂᑐᐦᑯᔮᓐᐦ ᑭᔮᐦ ᒫᒃ ᐊᓂᔮᐦ ᓂᑐᐦᑯᔮᓂᔅᐧᑳᐤᐦ ᔐᔥ ᓈᑖᐦ ᐧᐋᔥᑭᒡ ᒋᐱᐦ ᒌᐦ ᐧᐄᐦᑎᒫᑯ᙮

“ᔐᔥ ᐧᐄᐱᒡ ᒋᑭ ᓂᑎᐧᐋᔨᐦᑖᓐ ᒑ ᑖᐱᔑᒥᑭᐧᐃᔮᓐ ᒑ ᒌᐦ ᒥᐧᔮᑭᒥᐦᑖᑭᓂᐧᐃᒡ

ᒑᒃ ᒋᐹ ᒌᔒᐦᑲᒻ᙮

ᓇᒧᐃ ᒫᒃ ᐅᐦᒋ ᐊᔮᐤ ᒥᑖᐦᐧᑖᒋᒉᒥᑖᐦᑐᒥᑐᓅ᙮ ᑖᓂᑌ ᒫᒃ ᒋᐹᒌ ᐅᐦᒋ ᐊᔮᐤ ᐅᔫ ᔐᓚᔮᔫ ᐧᐁᔅ ᐁᑳ ᒌ ᐊᔮᑌ ᐊᓂᔫ ᒥᔅᑳᑎᐦᑳᓂᔫ ᐁᒄ ᑮᐹ ᓈᓂᑑ ᒦᓐ ᑫ ᒪᒋᔑᑲᓄᔭᒡ ᐊᓂᔫ ᐅᔅᑳᑦ ᒥᔫᓂᔭᒣ᙮ ᔐᓚᔮᔫᑲᒥᑯᐦᒡ ᑳ ᐃᑐᐦᑌᑦ ᓯᔅᑲᐦᐆᓈᐦᑎᒄᐦ ᐁ ᐋᐸᒋᐦᑖᑦ, ᑳ ᐅᐦᐋᓯᑦ ᔐᓚᔮᔫ ᑳ ᐅᑎᓂᒫᓯᑦ ᐊᓂᔫ ᑳ ᔐᓚᔮᐅᓂᔮᒡ ᒥᔅᑳᑎᐦᑳᓂᔫ᙮ ᒌᐧᐄ ᐋᔮᒥᐦᐄᑰ ᐅᔫ ᒥᒄ ᒫᒃ ᒌ ᒥᔦᔮᐦᑕᒻ ᐁᒌ ᐧᐄᒋᐦᐄᓯᑦ᙮ ᐃᔅᑯᑕᒃ ᒫᒃ ᑳ ᐃᔅᐧᑳᐤ ᑖᐱᐦᑕᑖᑲᓄᔭᒡ ᐊᓂᔫ ᒥᔅᑳᑎᐦᑳᓂᔫ ᑳ ᐅᔥᑳᔮᐤ, ᑳᐤ ᒌ ᒌᐧᐁᐤ, ᑳ ᐊᑎ ᐧᐊᐧᐁᔭᐱᑦ, ᑳ ᑌᐦᒋᔥᑖᑦ ᑖᐱᔅᑯᓐ ᐅᔅᑳᑦ ᒦᒋᓰᓈᐦᒋᑯᔑᐦᒡ ᐁᒄ ᑳ ᐲᔥᑌᐅᐸᔭᔑᐦᐧᑳᐤ ᑳ ᒥᓂᐦᐧᑫᑦ ᑫᒌ ᒋᔮᒣᐧᐁᔭᐦᑕᒃ᙮

ᐁᐅᒄ ᔮᐸᒡ ᒋᓯᓄ ᑳ ᐃᔑᓈᑯᓯᑦ ᐁ ᓰᐧᐋᑲᒥᐦᐧᑫᑦ ᑲᔦ ᐁ ᓃᐦᒋᐸᔭᐦᒡ ᐅᒥᐦᒄ ᐁ ᐋᐧᑫᔭᐦᑕᒃ ᐁᑳ ᑏᐧᐁᐦᒡ ᒌ ᐋᐱᔅᑯᔑᑦ, ᐋᐦᑯᓰᐅᑲᒥᑯᐦᒡ ᒌ ᑲᓇᐧᐁᔭᒫᑲᓅ ᒫᓐ ᐊᓂᔫ ᐁ ᐃᔅᐸᔭᑦ᙮ ᑫᒃ ᑳ ᒫᒥᑐᓄᔭᐦᑕᒃ ᐊᓂᔫ ᐁ ᒥᓂᐦᐧᑫᑦ, ᐁ ᐸᒋᔅᑲᐦᐆᓯᑦ ᐁᑯᑦ ᓯᔅᒋᑰᒡ ᑳ ᐅᐦᒋ ᐃᑌᔭᐦᑕᒃ ᐅᔫ ᒥᒄ ᒫᒃ ᒌ ᐃᑌᔭᐦᑕᒻ ᓈᓂᑑ ᓂᐹ ᐧᐄᐦᑕᒫᒄ ᓂᑐᐦᑯᐃᓐ ᒫᒃ ᓂᑐᐦᑯᐃᓂᔅᐧᑫᐤ᙮

ᑫᒃ ᐯᔭᐧᑳᐤ ᒌ ᐃᑎᑯ ᓂᑎᐦᑯᐃᓂᔅᐧᑫᐤ, “ᓂᑐᐧᐁᔭᐦᑖᑯᓐ ᒌᔅ ᑫᒌ ᑖᐱᔑᒥᑯᔭᓐ᙮ ᒌᔅ

Dix mille dollars, représentaient beaucoup plus d'argent que Jack n'en avait. Soit il trouvait cet argent, soit il se préparait à ce que le cycle d'infection-amputation ne recommence. Avec des béquilles, Jack alla à la banque, obtint un prêt et s'acheta la jambe artificielle dispendieuse. La situation était pénible – mais au moins, il avait pu faire quelque chose pour y remédier. Une fois la nouvelle jambe correctement ajutée, il rentra chez lui, posa ses deux jambes sur la table basse et but quelques bières pour se détendre.

Ten thousand dollars was a whole lot more money than Jack had. Either he had to come up with it or he had to get ready for the whole infection-amputation cycle to begin again. On crutches, Jack went to the bank, got a loan, and bought himself the expensive artificial leg. The situation was annoying – but at least he had been able to do something about it. After the new leg had been properly fitted, he went home, rested both legs on the coffee table and had a few beers to unwind.

Les comas diabétiques et hypoglycémiques, et les inévitables séjours à l'hôpital qui allaient avec, occupaient toujours une grande place dans la vie de Jack. Parfois, alors qu'il s'injectait de l'insuline, il se demandait si sa consommation d'alcool avait un rapport avec ces comas, mais si cela avait été le cas, un médecin ou une infirmière l'aurait sans aucun doute mentionné à un moment donné en cours de route.

Diabetic and hypoglycemic comas, and the inevitable hospital stays that came with them, were still a big part of Jack's life. Sometimes, as he injected himself with insulin, he wondered if his drinking had something to do with them, but surely, if that were the case, a doctor or nurse would have mentioned it somewhere along the way.

« Vous allez bientôt avoir besoin de dialyses, lui dit un jour une infirmière. Il

"You're going to need dialysis soon," a nurse said one day. "It's pretty clear that

ᒋᒥᐦᒄ," ᐄᑎᑰ ᐹᔩᐧᑳᐤ ᓂᑐᐦᑯᔨᓂᔅᐧᑳᐤᐦ᙮ "ᐛᔥ ᒌᐦᑳᓈᑯᓐ ᐋᑳ ᓈᔥᒡ ᒥᔪᐱᔨᔨᒡ ᐊᔥᑐᑎᐦᑯᓰᒡ᙮ ᐊᓂᑖᐦ ᐋ ᐧᒫᓐᑎᓅᐧᔩᑦ ᒋᑭ ᐄᔑ ᐋᐦᑎᐱᓐ ᐊᔥᑎᑖᔨᐦᑖᓐ᙮"

ᒥᒄ ᔩᑎᐤ ᐱᔮᐱᐦᐧᑳᔨᑦ ᒑᒃ, ᓂᒥ ᒋᔅᑐᑖᐤ᙮ ᐛᔥ ᐋ ᓂᒥ ᐧᐄᐦ ᒥᔪᓰᒡ ᓂᑐᑎᐦᑯᓰᒡ᙮ ᒌᐦ ᒋᔅᒑᔨᒫᐤ ᐊᐧᐋᔨᐤᐦ ᐋᐦ ᑖᐱᔑᒫᑭᓂᐧᐃᐧᐃᔨᒡᐦ᙮ ᒌᐦ ᒋᔅᒑᔨᐦᑎᒻ ᑭᔩᐦ ᐋᑳ ᐊᓂᔩ ᐧᐄᐦ ᐄᓯᓈᑯᓯᑦ ᐧᐄᔨ, ᐋᑳ ᑭᔨᐧᐹ ᓈᔥᒡ ᐊᐅᐧᐋᓐᐦ ᒑ ᒌᐦ ᐊᔨᐦᑎᒃ ᐊᓂᔩ ᐃᐦᑐᑎᐧᐋᑭᓂᐧᐃᒑ᙮ ᐊᓂᑖᐦ ᐧᐋᔥ ᐱᑯᑎᔅᑭᒥᑳᐦᒡ ᒌᐦ ᐧᐄᐦ ᐃᐦᑖᐤ᙮ ᒌᐦ ᐧᐄᐦ ᓂᑑᐦᐆ ᑭᔩᐦ ᒌᐦ ᐧᐄᐦ ᓅᑎᒫᓵᐤ᙮ ᒌᐦ ᐧᐄ ᐱᐹᐃᔨᐦᑖᐤ ᐊᓂᑖᐦ ᐄᔨᔨᐅᔅᒌᐦᒡ᙮ ᓂᒧᐃ ᐅᐦᒋ ᓂᑎᐧᐋᔨᐦᑎᒻ ᒑ ᑖᐱᔑᒫᑭᓂᐧᐃᑦ᙮

ᐄᔅᑯᑎᒃ ᒫᒃ ᑳ ᐄᔑᓈᑯᓂᔨᒡ ᒑ ᒌᐦ ᐃᐦᑐᑎᐦᒃ, ᒑᒃ ᒌᐦ ᓈᓂᑑᒋᔅᒑᔨᐦᑎᒻ ᑖᓂᑖᐦ ᒦᓐ ᒑ ᒌᐦ ᐃᐦᑎᒃ ᐄᔥᐱᔑᐧᐄ ᒑ ᑖᐱᔑᒫᑭᓂᐧᐃᑦ ᓂᑐᐧᐋᐱᐦᒋᑭᓂᔨᐤ ᐋᐦ ᐋᐱᒋᔥᑖᑦ᙮ ᑳ ᒥᔅᑭᐦᒃ = ᑭᔩᐦ ᑳ ᐄᔑᓈᑯᓂᔨᒡ ᓈᔥᒡ ᐋᐦᐧᑳᒡ, ᐧᒫᐦᒡ ᐊᓂᔩ ᑳ ᒥᓂᔑᑭᓂᐧᐃᐧᐃᔨᒡ ᐅᔅᑳᑦ᙮ ᒋᑭ ᒌᐦ ᒥᓂᐧᐛᑭᓂᐧᐃᐧᐃᔨᐤᐦ ᐅᑐᑎᐦᑯᓯᐤᐦ ᑭᔩᐦ ᒋᑭ ᒌᐦ ᒥᔩᑭᓂᐤ ᑯᑎᒃᐦ᙮ ᑭᔩᐦ ᐋᑯᑖᐦ ᒑ ᒌᐦ ᐃᐦᑐᑎᐧᐋᑭᓂᐧᐃᑦ ᐊᓂᔩᐦ ᒫᐧᑳᒡ ᐋᐦ ᒦᔥᑯᑎᒧᐦᐧᐋᑭᓂᐧᐃᐧᐃᔨᒡᐦ ᐅᐲᔥᐲᔥᒃᐦ ᐊᓂᔩ ᑭᔨᐧᐹ ᐋᑳ ᒌᐦ ᐃᐦᑎᔨᒡᐦ ᐊᓂᔩᐦ ᒫᐧᑳᒡ ᐋᔩᐧᐋᑦ᙮ ᒨᔥ ᑳᐦ ᐄᑖᑭᓂᐧᐃᑦ ᐋᑳ ᓂᐦᑖ ᒑ ᒌᐦ ᓂᑭᑎᑯᑦ ᐊᐧᐋᓐ ᒥᔑᐤ ᐋᐦ ᐛᑳᐅᐱᔨᑦ᙮ ᑳᐦ ᐄᑎᑯᑦ ᐊᓂᔩᐦ ᓂᑐᐦᑯᔨᓐ ᒥᔑᐤ ᐋ ᐃᔩᒡᐦ ᐊᐧᐋᓐ ᐊᓂᔩ ᐋᐦᑯᓯᐧᐃᓂᔨᐤ ᒑ ᐄᔥᐱᔑ ᐱᒫᑎᓰᑦ ᑭᑎ ᐃᔩᐤ᙮ ᒥᒄ ᒫᒃ ᒌᐦ

ᓇᒧᐃ ᐃᔅᐱᔅ ᒥᔫᐛᐤ ᒋᑌᐦᑕᑯᓰᐤ᙮ ᒋᑲᒌ ᐋᐦᑐᑫᓐ ᐋ ᒨᓄᔩᐦᐤ ᒋᑎᑌᔨᐦᑌᓐ"᙮

ᒌ ᐹᐦᐱᐦᐧᑫᔨᔥᑐᐧᐁᐤ ᒥᒄ ᓇᒧᐃ ᑫᐧᑳᔫ ᐅᐦᒋ ᐃᑌᐤ᙮ ᓂᑌᐦᑕᑯᓰᐤ ᐋ, ᒌ ᐃᑌᔨᐦᑕᒻ᙮ ᒌ ᒋᔅᑫᔨᒣᐤ ᐊᐧᐁᔫᐦ ᐁ ᑖᐱᔑᒫᑲᓅᔨᒡ᙮ ᒌ ᐧᐋᐸᒣᐤ ᐁᑳ ᓈᔅᒡ ᒌ ᐃᐦᑑᑕᒥᔨᒡ ᑫᐧᑳᔫ ᓇᒧᐃ ᐅᐦᒋ ᐧᐄ ᐃᔑᓈᑯᓰ ᐧᐄ᙮ ᒌᐧᐄ ᐃᐦᑖᐤ ᓅᐦᒋᒦᐦᒡ᙮ ᒌᐧᐄ ᓂᑑᐦᐆ ᑲᔦ ᒋᐧᐄ ᓅᑕᒣᓴᐤ᙮ ᒌᐧᐄ ᐸᐹ ᐊᐃᐦᑖᐤ ᐄᓅ ᐊᔅᒌᐦᒡ᙮ ᑖᐱᔑᒫᑲᓅᑦ ᓇᒧᐃ ᒋᐹᒌ ᐃᐦᑑ ᐊᓂᔫ ᐧᐋ ᐃᐦᑎᑦ ᐧᐄ᙮

ᐁᒄ ᐃᔅᑯᑕᒃ ᓀᐦᐄᐸᔨᑦ ᒌ ᓈᓂᑑ ᒋᔅᑫᔨᐦᑕᒻ ᐁ ᐃᐦᑕᑯᓂᔨᐧᑫ ᒦᓐ ᑖᓐ ᑫᒌ ᐃᐦᑎᑦ ᐊᓂᔫ ᐁᑳ ᓂᑐᐧᐁᔨᐦᑕᐦᒃ ᑫᒌ ᑖᐱᔑᒫᑲᓅᑦ᙮ ᑫᒃ ᑳ ᒥᔅᑲᐦᒃ ᐯᔭᒄ ᑫᐧᑳᔫ ᑫᒌ ᐃᐦᑎᑦ = ᒥᒄ ᒫᒃ ᐯᔭᑯᓂᐦᒡ ᒋᐹ ᐃᑌᔨᐦᑖᑯᓂᔫ ᑖᓐ ᑳ ᐃᔅᐸᔨᑦ ᑳ ᒋᒪᓯᑲᓂᔨᒡ ᐅᔅᑳᑦ᙮ ᒋᐱᒌ ᒪᓂᐧᓵᑲᓅᔫ ᐯᔭᒄ ᐅᑌᐦᑕᑯᓰ ᐁᒄ ᑯᑕᒃ ᒋᐹ ᒋᑲᒧᐦᐧᐋᑲᓅᔫᐦ ᐊᓂᑕ᙮ ᒫᒃ ᑲᔦ, ᐊᓂᔫ ᒣᐧᑳᒡ ᐃᐦᑑᑐᐧᐋᑲᓅᑦ, ᐊᓂᔫ ᐅᐦᐹᐱᑯᓰᒻ ᐁᑳ ᓵᔅ ᑳ ᒥᔫᓯᔨᒡ ᑯᑕᒃ ᒋᐱᐦᒌ ᒋᑲᒧᐦᐧᐋᑲᓅᔫ ᐊᓂᑕ᙮ ᒨᔥ ᐁᑯᓐ ᑳᒌ ᐯᒋ ᐃᑎᑯᑦ ᓂᑐᐦᑯᐃᓐ ᐁᑳ ᐃᐦᑕᑯᐦᒡ ᑫᒌᔑ ᒦᓂᐧᐋᒋᐦᐧᐋᑲᓅᑦ ᐊᐧᐁᓐ ᑳ ᓰᐧᐋᑲᒥᐦᐧᑫᑦ᙮ ᐊᐧᐁᓐ ᑳ ᓰᐧᐋᑲᒥᐸᔨᑦ ᒨᔥ ᒋᑲ ᓰᐧᐋᑲᒥᐸᔫ᙮ ᒥᒄ ᒫᒃ ᒌ ᐃᑌᔨᐦᑕᒻ, ᐅᔅᒋᓰᑦ ᓅᐦᐹᐱᑯᓰᐤ, ᐁᑳ ᐅᐦᒋ ᐧᐊᓈᑎᓰᑦ ᓰᐧᐋᑲᒥᐦᐧᑫᐧᐃᓂᔫ ᐅᐦᒋ, ᒋᑲᒌ ᐃᔑᓈᑯᓂᔫ ᑖᐧᐯ ᒋᐦᒋᐧᐁ ᑫᒌ ᒦᓂᐧᐋᑎᓰᑦ᙮

est assez évident que vos reins lâchent. Pensez-vous que déménagerez-vous à Montréal dans ce cas ? »

your kidneys are giving out. Will you be moving to Montréal, then, do you think?"

Jack lui sourit poliment mais ne répondit pas. Ses reins ? Il connaissait des gens sous dialyse. Leurs vies étaient beaucoup plus limitées que ce qu'il ne voudrait jamais pour lui-même. Il avait besoin de pouvoir aller dans le bois. Il devait pouvoir chasser et pêcher. Il devait pouvoir se déplacer autour de l'Eeyou Istchee. La dialyse n'était tout simplement pas une option.

Jack smiled politely but didn't answer. His kidneys? He knew people on dialysis. Their lives were much more restricted than he wanted ever to be. He needed to be able to go to the bush. He needed to be able to hunt and fish. He needed to be able to move around Eeyou Istchee. Dialysis simply was not an option.

Dès qu'il en fut capable, Jack commença à chercher sur Internet pour trouver d'autres options que la dialyse. Il en trouva une - et elle était tout aussi radicale que l'amputation. Un de ses reins pourrait être enlevé et remplacé par un rein transplanté. En même temps, son pancréas épuisé pourrait être remplacé un pancréas transplanté. Les médecins lui avaient toujours dit qu'il n'y avait aucun remède contre le diabète. Diabétique un jour, diabétique toujours. Toutefois, s'il recevait un nouveau pancréas, qui ne serait pas épuisé par le diabète, il y aurait une chance qu'il soit vraiment guéri.

As soon as he was able, Jack began looking online for options other than dialysis. He found one – and it was every bit as drastic as amputation. He could have his kidney cut out and replaced with a transplanted kidney. He could also, at the same time, have his burnt-out pancreas replaced with a transplanted one. The doctors had always told him that there was no cure for diabetes. Once diabetic, always diabetic. But if he got a new pancreas, one not burnt out by diabetes, there was a chance that he might truly be cured.

ᒥᔮᑭᓂᐧᐃᒑ ᑯᑎᒃᐦ ᐅᐲᔥᐲᔥᒃᐦ ᐋᐦ ᒥᔪᓯᔭᒡᐦ ᐋᑯᑎᐦ ᒋᔥᒋᐧᐋ ᒑ ᒌᐦ ᐅᐦᒋ ᒦᓂᐧᐋᑎᓰᑦ᙮

ᒦᓐ ᒫᒃ ᐊᓂᑖᐦ ᑳ ᓂᑑᑎᐹᔮᒪᑭᓂᐧᐃᑦ ᐧᒫᓐᑎᓅᐧᔮᑦ, ᑳᐦ ᑯᐧᑳᒋᒫᑦ ᒑᒃ ᓂᑐᐦᑯᔮᓐᐦ ᐊᓂᔮ ᐋᐦ ᒦᔥᑯᑎᒧᐦᑖᑭᓂᐧᐃᐧᐃᔭᒡ ᐊᐧᐋᓐ ᒑᐧᑳᔭᐤ ᐲᐦᒡ ᐅᔮᐦᒡ᙮

“ᑖᐧᐹ ᒑᒃ, ᐄᑎᑰ ᐊᓂᔮᐦ ᓂᑐᐦᑯᔮᓐᐦ, ᑭᔭᐧᐹ ᐋᑖᔭᐦᑎᒫᓐ ᐊᓐ ᒑ ᒌᐦ ᒦᔪᐱᔭᐦᐄᑯᔭᓐ ᐃᐦᑐᑖᑭᐧᐃᔭᓈ᙮ ᐋᔪᐧᐃᒄ ᑭᔭᐧᐹ ᐋᐦ ᐃᐦᑐᑎᐧᐋᑭᓂᐅᐧᐃᒡ ᑯᑎᑭᒡ ᐊᐧᐋᓂᒌ᙮ ᐋᐅᒄ ᑭᔭᐧᐹ ᒦᓐ ᐊᓐ ᒑ ᒌᐦ ᑯᒋᔥᑖᔭᓐ ᐋᐦ ᑖᐱᔑᒥᑭᐧᐃᐧᐃᔭᓐ᙮ ᒥᐧᔮᔭᐤ ᐧᐋᔥ ᐊᓂᔮ ᐋᐦ ᐄᐦᑐᑎᐧᐋᑭᓂᐧᐃᑦ ᐊᐧᐋᓐ᙮ ᒥᐦᒑᑐ ᐊᐧᐋᓂᒌ ᐅᑎᐦ ᐃᐦᑐᑎᐧᐋᑭᓂᐅᐧᐃᒡ”᙮

ᒥᒄ ᐱᔮᐦᐱᐦᐧᑳᔭᑦ ᒑᒃ = ᓈᑖᐦ ᐋᔅᐱᔭᑦ ᐊᓂᑖᐦ ᓂᑐᐦᑯᔭᓂᑭᒥᑯᐦᒡ ᐋᐦ ᒦᔥᑯᑎᒧᐦᑖᑭᓂᐧᐃᐧᐃᔭᒡ ᐲᐦᒡ ᐅᔮᐧᐋᐦᒡ ᒑᐧᑳᔭᐤ ᐊᐧᐋᓂᒌ, ᐋᑯᑎᐦ ᒥᒄ ᐋᔥᐱᔒᑦ ᐋᐦ ᑯᐧᑳᒋᔅᒑᒧᑦ ᐊᓂᔮ ᒑᐧᑳᔭᐤ ᐧᐋᐦ ᒋᔅᒑᔭᐦᑎᐦᒃ᙮ ᐊᐧᑳᑖᑭᓂᐧᐃᑦ ᐋᐦᐧᒫᔮᐦ ᒌᐦ ᒫᒥᑐᓈᔭᐦᑎᒥᐦᐄᐧᐋᔭᒡ ᐊᓂᔮ ᒑ ᒌᐦ ᐃᐦᑐᑎᐧᐋᑭᓂᐧᐃᑦ ᐱᑎᒫ ᐊᑎᑎᐤ ᒋᑭ ᐧᐄᐦ ᒦᓂᐧᐋᒋᐦᐋᑭᓂᐆ ᐅᐦᒋ ᐊᓂᔮ ᐋᐦ ᔔᑳᐅᐱᔭᑦ ᑭᔮᐦ ᓈᔥᒡ ᑯᐃᔅᒄ ᒑ ᓈᓈᑭᒋᐦᑖᑦ ᐊᓂᔮ ᐋᔑ ᒦᒋᓯᑦ᙮ ᐊᓂᔮ ᒫᒃ ᐊᑎᑎᐤ ᒐ ᐋᔭᒥᔭᑯᑦ ᐋᔪᐧᐃᒄ ᓈᔥᑎᔭᒡ ᒐ ᐴᓃᑦ ᐋᐦ ᒥᓂᐦᐧᑳᑦ᙮ ᒌᐦ ᐄᐦᑐᑎᐦᑲ ᒫᒃ ᐅᔮᐦ ᓃᔓ ᒑᐧᑳᔭᐤᐦ ᐧᑳᐧᔔᓐ ᐋᑯᑎᐦ ᒑ ᒌᐦ ᐄᔑᓈᑯᓂᔭᒡ ᒐ ᒌᐦ ᐃᐦᑐᑎᐧᐋᑭᓂᐧᐃᑦ ᐊᓂᔮ ᐋᔑ ᑯᐧᑳᒋᔅᒑᒧᑦ᙮ ᒌᐦ ᐃᐦᑐᑎᐦᑲ ᒫᒃ

ᐁᒄ ᑮᐹ ᒦᓐ ᑳ ᓂᑐᐧᐋᐸᒫᑦ ᓂᑐᐦᑯᐃᓐ ᐊᓂᑌ ᒨᓭᔮᐦᒡ, ᑳ ᑲᐧᑫᒋᒫᑦ ᑖᓐ ᐁ ᐃᐦᑎᑦ ᐊᐧᐁᓐ ᐁ ᓂᑐᐧᐁᔭᐦᑕᐦᒃ ᑫᒌ ᐅᔅᑳᔭᒡ ᑫᐧᑳᔫ ᐊᓂᑕ ᐲᐦᒌᔫ ᐁ ᐃᐦᑖᑦ ᐁᑳ ᓵᔅ ᒥᐧᔮᔭᒡ ᐊᓂᔫ ᐧᐄ ᑳ ᐋᔮᑦ᙮

“ᓇᒧᐃ”, ᒌ ᐃᑎᑰ, “ᓇᒧᐃ ᒋᑲᒌ ᐃᔑᓈᑯᓐ ᒌᔭ ᑫᒌ ᐃᐦᑑᑖᑯᔭᓐ᙮ ᑯᑕᑲᒡ ᐊᐧᐁᓐ ᒋᑲᒌ ᐃᐦᑑᑕᐧᐋᑲᓅᒡ᙮ ᑯᒋᐦᑖ ᑫᒌ ᑖᐱᔑᒥᑯᔭᓐ᙮ ᒋᑲ ᐧᐄᒋᐦᐄᑰᓐ ᐧᐁᓯᓐ ᑖᐱᔑᒥᑯᔭᓀ᙮ ᒥᐦᑫᑑᒡ ᐊᐧᐁᓂᒌ ᐅᑕᐦ ᐁ ᑖᐱᔑᒫᑲᓅᐧᑖᐤ”᙮

ᑳ ᐹᐦᐱᐦᐧᑫᔥᑐᐧᐋᑦ ᐊᓂᔫᐦ ᓂᑐᐦᑯᐃᓐᐦ = ᐁᒄ ᓀᑌ ᑳ ᐊᑎ ᐃᔅᐸᔭᑦ ᐊᓂᑌ ᒥᔮᑎᐧᔔᑲᓅᐧᑖᐤ ᐊᐧᐁᓂᒌ ᐁ ᓂᑐᐧᐁᔭᐦᑖᑯᓂᔭᒡ ᑫᒌ ᒪᓂᔑᑲᓄᔭᒡ ᐊᓂᔫ ᐁᑳ ᑳ ᒥᐧᔮᔭᒡ ᑫᐧᑳᔫ ᐊᓂᑕ ᐲᐦᒋᔫ ᐁ ᐃᐦᑖᑦ ᐁᒄ ᑯᑕᒋᐦᔫ ᑫᑲᒧᐦᑖᑲᓄᔭᒡ ᐊᓂᑕᐦ, ᓇᓈᐦᑰ ᒌᔑ ᑲᐧᑫᒋᐦᑫᔭᒨ ᐁᐧᐄ ᓂᑑ ᒋᔅᑫᔭᐦᑕᐦᒃ ᐅᔫ᙮ ᐊᓂᔫᐦ ᒫᒃ ᐊᐧᐁᔫᐦ ᐊᓂᑕ ᑳ ᐋᐸᑎᓯᔭᒡ ᐁ ᓂᑑ ᒋᔅᑫᔭᒫᐧᑖᐤ ᐊᐧᐁᔫᐦ ᑫ ᓂᑐᐧᐁᔭᐦᑖᑯᓂᔭᐧᑫ ᑫᒌ ᒫᑎᐧᔔᑲᓄᔭᒡ ᒌ ᐄᑎᑰ ᐱᑕᒫ ᑫᒌ ᓇᓈᑲᑐᐧᐁᔭᐦᑕᐦᒃ ᐊᓂᔫ ᐁ ᔔᑳᐅᐸᔭᑦ ᐁᑎᑑ ᑫᒌ ᒥᔫᐸᔭᔭᒡ ᑲᔦ ᑫᒌ ᒦᒋᑦ ᒦᒋᒥᔫ ᐁ ᒥᔫᔅᑳᑫᒪᑲᓂᔭᒡ᙮ ᑲᔦ ᒫᒃ ᑫᒌ ᐴᓃᑦ ᐁ ᒥᓂᐦᐧᑫᑦ, ᐁᐅᒄ ᒫᐅᒡ ᒋᐹ ᐋᔭᒥᐦᐄᑰ ᒑᒃ ᑫᒌ ᐃᐦᑎᑦ ᒌ ᐃᑌᔭᐦᑕᒻ᙮

Lors de sa visite de contrôle suivante à Montréal, Jack interrogea le médecin à propos des organes transplantés.

« Oh Jack. Je ne pense pas que vous soyez un bon candidat pour ça, lui répondit le médecin. C'est plutôt une solution pour... d'autres personnes. Cependant, vous pourriez essayer la dialyse. Ce n'est pas si mal, vous savez. Beaucoup de gens ici y ont recours ».

Jack lui sourit poliment – puis traversa la ville en voiture pour se rendre à la clinique de transplantation, où il posa question après question. Avant même que les chirurgiens ne l'envisagent pour une transplantation, les gens de la clinique lui dirent, Jack devrait mieux contrôler son diabète et manger régulièrement une alimentation saine. Plus difficile encore, il devrait arrêter de boire complètement. S'il parvenait à atteindre ces deux objectifs, il serait peut-être éligible. S'il était éligible, il serait inscrit sur une liste. Ensuite, il devrait attendre de voir si une personne dont les tissus seraient

At his next check-up in Montréal, Jack asked the doctor about transplanted organs.

"Oh Jack. I don't think you'd be a good candidate for that," the doctor said. "That's more a solution for – other people. But you could try dialysis. It's not so bad, you know. Lots of folks around here do it."

Jack smiled politely – then drove across town to the transplant clinic, where he asked question after question. Before transplant surgeons would even consider him for a transplant, the people at the clinic said, Jack would have to have his diabetes under better control and be regularly eating a healthy diet. Even harder, he would have to stop drinking altogether. If he managed to do those two things, then he might be eligible. If he was eligible, he'd be put on a list. After that, he would have to wait and see if anyone with healthy matching tissues died and donated her or his organs to

ᐅᔮ ᐋᐦ ᓃᔑᓂᔨᒡ ᒑ ᐱᒋᔅᑎᓂᑭᓂᐧᐃᐧᐃᔨᒡ ᐅᑎᓯᓂᐦᑳᓲᐧᐃᓐ ᒑ ᒌᐦ ᒥᔮᑭᓂᐧᐃᑦ ᑯᑎᒋᔨᐤ ᐊᓂᔮ ᒑᐧᑳᔨᐤ ᓈᑎᐧᐋᔨᐦᑎᐦᒃ. ᐄᔅᑯᑎᒃ ᒫᒃ ᒌᐦ ᒥᓯᓂᐦᐧᐋᑭᓂᐧᐃᒑ, ᒥᒄ ᒑ ᐋᓯᓂᐧᐋᓯᑦ ᒑ ᐃᐦᑖᔨᐧᑳᓂᐦᐄ ᐊᐧᐋᔨᐤᐦ ᓈᐦᐋᐤ ᐊᓂᔮᐦ ᐋᐦ ᐄᔑ ᐃᔮᔨᐦᒡ ᐋᔑᔮᑦ ᐊᓂᑖᐦ ᐲᐦᒋᔨᐤ, ᒑ ᒌᐦ ᓂᐦᐄᔥᑳᑯᑦ ᑭᔨᐧᐹ, ᐊᓂᔮᐦ ᑭᔨᐧᐸ ᐊᐧᐋᔨᐤᐦ ᐋᐦ ᐱᒋᔅᑎᓂᒥᔨᒡᐦ ᒑ ᒌᐦ ᐋᐱᑎᓂᔨᒡᐦ ᐄᔅᑯᑎᒃ ᐴᓂᐱᒫᑎᓯᔨᐧᑖᐧᐋᓂᐦᐄ. ᒥᔮᑭᓂᐧᐃᒑ ᒫᒃ ᒑᒃ ᐊᓂᔮ ᐋᔑ ᓂᑎᐧᐋᔨᐦᑎᐦᒃ ᓂᑐᐦᑯᔨᓐᐦ ᒋᑭ ᐅᑎᓂᒻ ᑮᔮᐦ ᒨᔥ ᒋᑭ ᔖᔕᐧᐄᐤ ᑮᔮᐦ ᑯᐃᔅᒄ ᒋᑭ ᒦᒋᓲ ᑮᔮᐦ ᓂᒥ ᓂᐦᑖ ᒋᑭ ᒥᓂᐦᐧᑳᐤ ᑮᔮᐦ ᓂᒥ ᓂᐦᑖ ᑭᑎ ᐋᐱᒋᐦᑖᐤ ᒥᒋᓂᑐᐦᑯᔨᓐᐦ. ᓈᔥᑖᐧᐹ ᒥᔥᒌᐦ ᑭᑎ ᐧᐄᐦ ᐄᔑ ᐋᐦᒋᔥᑖᐤ ᐅᐱᒫᑎᓲᐧᐃᓐ ᑮᔮᐦ ᒫᒃ ᒋᑭ ᒌᐦ ᐄᔑᓈᑯᓂᔨᐤ ᐋᑳ ᒑ ᒌᐦ ᒥᔮᑭᓂᐧᐃᑦ ᐋᐦ ᓂᐦᐄᔥᑳᑯᑦ ᐋᑦ ᐅᔭ ᒥᓯᐧᐊ ᐊᑎ ᐃᔨᐦᑎᒐ. ᒥᒄ ᒫᒃ ᐊᔭᐱᒡ ᑭᑎ ᑯᒋᔥᑖᐤ. ᓈᔥᑖᐧᐹᐦ ᔖᔥ ᔑᔥᑭᒋᐦᐄᑰ ᒥᒄ ᐋᐦ ᐄᔑ ᑭᑭᐧᐃᐦᑯᔑᑦ ᑮᔮᐦ ᐋᐦ ᐋᐦᑯᓭᐹᐧᐋᑦ. ᔖᔥ ᓈᔥᑎᔨᒡ ᓂᒥ ᓯᓭᐱᐦᐄᑰ ᐅᔮ ᒑ ᒌᐦ ᐄᔑ ᐃᐦᑐᑎᐦᒃ.

ᑳᐦ ᐴᓃᑦ ᒑᒃ ᐋᐦ ᒥᓂᐦᐧᑳᑦ ᑮᔮᐦ ᒥᒋᓂᑐᐦᑯᔨᓐᐦ ᐋᐦ ᐋᐱᒋᐦᑖᑦ. ᓈᔥᒡ ᐋᐦ ᒌᐦ ᐋᔨᒥᐦᐄᑯᑦ ᐅᔮ ᒑ ᒌᐦ ᐃᐦᑐᑎᐦᒃ. ᐋᔨᒋᒑ ᒫᐅᒡ ᑳᐦ ᐋᔨᒥᐦᐄᑯᑦ ᒑᐧᑳᔨᐤ ᐋᐦ ᐧᐄᐦ ᐃᐦᑐᑎᐦᒃ. ᓂᒥᒌᐧᐋ ᐅᐦᒋ ᐄᑐᐦᑕᐤ ᐊᓂᑖᐦ ᐋᐦ ᓂᔥᑎᐧᐄᓈᓂᐧᐃᐧᐃᔨᒡ ᐋᐦ ᐧᐄᐦ ᐴᓃᓈᓂᐧᐃᔨᒡ ᐋᐦ ᒥᓂᐦᐧᑳᓂᐧᐃᐧᐃᔨᒡ ᑮᔮᐦ ᒥᒋᓂᑐᐦᑯᔨᓐᐦ ᐋᐦ ᐴᓂᐦᑖᑭᓂᐧᐃᐧᐃᔨᒡᐦ

ᒌ ᐃᐦᑑᑕᐦᐧᑫ ᒫᒃ ᐅᔦᐦ ᓃᓴ ᑫᐧᑳᔦ ᐁ ᐃᑕᓴᒫᑲᓅᑦ ᐁᒄ ᔮᒄ ᒋᐹᒌ ᐃᔑᓈᑯᓂᔦ ᑫᒌ ᒫᒋᐧᔖᑲᓅᑦ ᒌ ᐄᑖᑲᓅ. ᐁᒄ ᒫᒃ ᔮᒄ ᒋᐹ ᐊᔑᑎᓯᓇᐦᐧᐋᑲᓅ ᑲᔦ ᐧᐃᔮ ᒣ ᒫᒋᐧᔖᑲᓅᑦ. ᐁᒄ ᒫᒃ ᒥᒄ ᒋᐹ ᐊᓴᐧᐋᐴ ᒣᒌ ᐧᐄᔖᒫᑲᓅᑦ ᐃᔅᑯᑕᒃ ᐃᐦᑕᑯᓂᔨᒣ ᐊᓂᔦ ᓀᑐᐧᐁᔨᐦᑕᐦᒃ ᐁᒌ ᓂᐱᔨᒡ ᐊᐧᐁᔦ ᒣᒌ ᐅᐦᑎᓂᑲᓄᔨᒡ, ᐁᒌ ᐃᐧᑌᔨᒡ ᒣᒌ ᒪᓂᔑᑲᓄᔨᒡ ᐊᓂᑕ ᐁ ᐃᐦᑖᑦ ᒣᐧᔮᔨᑫ ᒫᒃ ᑯᑕᒃ ᐊᐧᐁᔦ ᒣᒌ ᐊᔮᔨᒡ. ᑖᐧᐯ ᒫᒃ ᒌ ᐃᐦᑑᑐᐧᐋᑲᓅᑌ ᐅᔦ ᐁᒄ ᒋᐹ ᐅᑎᓇᒻ ᓂᑐᐦᑯᐃᓐᐦ ᑲᔦ ᒨᔥ ᒋᐹ ᓭᓭᐅᐸᔦᐦᐆ, ᑲᔦ ᒨᔥ ᐁ ᒥᔦᔅᑳᒣᒪᑲᓂᔨᒡ ᒦᒋᒥᔦ ᒋᐹ ᒦᒎ ᓀᔅᑕ ᑲᔦ ᓇᒧᐃ ᒦᓐ ᐧᐄᔅᑳᑦ ᒋᐹ ᐅᐦᒋ ᒥᓂᐦᐧᑫᐤ ᐃᔅᑯᑌᐧᐋᐴᔦ ᑲᔦ ᒫᒃ ᓇᒧᐃ ᒦᓐ ᐧᐄᔅᑳᒡ ᒋᐹ ᐅᐦᒋ ᐅᑎᓇᒻ ᒪᒋᓂᑐᐦᑯᐃᓂᔦ. ᐁᐅᒄ ᐅᔦ ᒋᐹ ᐃᔑ ᓇᓈᑲᒋᐦᑖᐤ ᒣ ᐃᔥ ᐱᔥ ᐱᒫᑎᓲᐧᑫ. ᑖᐧᐯ ᑮᐹ ᒋᐹ ᐋᔨᒥᐦᐄᑰ ᒣᒌ ᐃᐦᑑᑕᐦᒃ ᐅᔦ ᑲᔦ ᒋᐱᒌ ᐃᔑᓈᑯᓂᔦ ᐁᑳ ᒥᔅᑳᑲᓄᔨᒡ ᐊᓂᔦ ᓀᑐᐧᐁᔨᐦᑕᐦᒃ ᐲᐦᒌᔦ ᒣᒌ ᐊᔮᑦ ᐁ ᐅᔅᑳᔨᒡ, ᐁᒌ ᓂᐱᔨᒡ ᐊᐧᐁᔦᐦ ᐧᐃᔦᐧᐃᔨᐦᒡ ᐁᒌ ᐅᐦᒋ ᒪᓂᔑᑲᓄᔨᒡ. ᒌᐧᐃ ᑯᒋᐦᑖᐤ ᒫᒃ ᔮᐸᒡ ᒣᒌ ᐃᐦᑑᑕᐦᒃ ᑖᓐ ᐁ ᐃᑕᓴᒫᑲᓅᑦ. ᓭᔅ ᑮᐹ ᒥᔑᐧᐋᒡ ᒌ ᓭᔅᑲᒋᐦᐄᑰ ᒨᔥ ᐁ ᐋᐦᑯᓯᑦ ᑲᔦ ᒨᔥ ᐁ ᐋᐦᑯᓯᐧᐋᐹᐧᐁᑦ. ᓭᔅ ᐧᐁᔅᑲᒡ ᐁᑳ ᑳ ᒋᐦᑳᐧᐋᑌᔨᒧᐦᐄᑯᑦ ᐅᔦ ᐁ ᐃᔅᐸᔨᑦ.

ᑳ ᐴᓃᑦ ᐁ ᒥᓂᐦᐧᑫᑦ ᑲᔦ ᒌ ᐴᓂᐦᑖᐤ ᒪᒋᓂᑐᐦᑯᐃᓐᐦ. ᓇᒧᐃ ᒫᒃ ᒥᒍᓐ ᐅᐦᒋ ᐧᐁᐦᒋᐦᐄᑰ. ᐁᐅᒄ ᐅᔦ ᒫᐅᒡ ᑳ ᐋᔨᒥᐦᐄᑯᑦ ᒣᐧᑳᔦ ᒣᒌ ᐃᐦᑑᑕᐦᒃ. ᓇᒧᐃ ᐅᐦᒋ ᐃᑐᐦᑌᐤ ᐊᓂᑌ ᐧᐁᐦᒋ ᐧᐄᒋᐦᐋᑲᓅᐧᑖᐤ ᑳ ᐧᐄᒋᐯᐧᑖᐤ ᑲᔦ ᑳ ᐧᐄᐦᒋᒪᒋᓂᑐᐦᑯᐦᐄᓯᐧᑖᐤ ᐧᐁᔅ ᑖᐹ ᐁᔅᒄ ᐅᐦᒋ ᐃᐦᑑᑖᑲᓅ ᐆ ᐊᓂᑌ ᐧᐋᔅᐧᐊᓂᐲᐦᒡ

sains et compatibles décédait en faisant don de ses organes à des personnes qui en auraient besoin. Si Jack recevait les organes, il devrait prendre des pilules spéciales, faire de l'exercice, manger sainement et ne pas boire d'alcool ni se droguer pour le reste de sa vie. Ce serait beaucoup de travail et peut-être qu'au final il n'y aurait aucun organe pour lui. Toutefois, il pouvait essayer. Quoi qu'il en soit, il commençait à en avoir assez des comas et des gueules de bois. Ceux-ci avaient perdu leur attrait depuis longtemps déjà.

people who needed them. If Jack got the organs, he would have to take special pills and he'd have to exercise and eat healthy and never drink alcohol and never get high for the rest of his life. It would be a big big deal and maybe in the end there would be no organs for him. But he could try. And he was getting pretty tired of comas and hangovers anyways. They had lost their appeal a long time ago.

Jack arrêta de boire et de se droguer. Ce n'était pas facile du tout. C'était probablement la chose la plus difficile qu'il ait jamais faite. Il ne fréquentait aucun groupe des Alcooliques Anonymes ou des Narcotiques Anonymes – Waswanipi n'avait pas de tels groupes à l'époque – et

Jack quit drinking and he quit doing drugs. It was not easy at all. It was probably the hardest thing he had ever done. He attended no Alcoholics Anonymous nor Narcotics Anonymous group – Waswanipi had no such groups back then – and he had no support

= ᓂᒧᐃ ᐅᐦᒋ ᐃᐦᑎᑯᓂᔨᐤ ᐅᔮ ᐊᓂᑖᐦ ᐧᐋᐧᓵᓂᐲᐦᒡ = ᓈᔥᑎᔨᒡ ᓂᒥ ᐅᐦᒋ ᐃᐦᑎᑯᓂᔨᐤ ᐊᓂᑖᐦ ᒑ ᒌᐦ ᐅᐦᒋ ᔒᑐᔥᑭᐧᐋᑭᓂᐧᐃᑦ᙮ ᑭᔮᐦ ᐋᔭᐧᐃᒄ ᑳᐦ ᐃᐦᑐᑎᐦᒃ ᐋᑳ ᒑ ᒌᐦ ᐱᐹᐧᐄᒑᐧᐋᑦ ᐊᓂᔮᐦ ᐅᐧᐄᒑᐧᐋᑭᓐᐦ ᓈᔥᒡ ᑳᐦ ᓵᒋᐦᐋᑦ ᐋᑦ ᓈᔥᒡ ᑭᔨᐧᐹ ᒌᐦ ᒥᐧᔮᔨᒫᑦ᙮ ᐊᓂᑖᐦ ᐧᐋᒑᐧᐋᒡᐦ ᓈᔥᒡ ᐋᐦ ᒌᐦ ᒫᑯᐦᐄᑯᑦ ᐋᐦ ᐧᐄᐦ ᒥᓂᐦᐧᑳᑦ᙮ ᐋᔭᐧᐃᒄ ᑭᔨᐧᐹ ᑳ ᐄᔑ ᒋᐢᒑᔨᐦᑎᐦᒃ ᐋᑳ ᒥᓂᐦᐧᑳᒑ ᑭᔮᐦ ᐋᑳ ᐋᐱᒋᐦᑖᒑ ᒥᒋᓂᑐᐦᑯᐃᓐᐦ ᐋᑯᑎᐦ ᓂᒥ ᑭᑎ ᑖᐱᔑᒫᑭᓂᐆ ᒑ ᒌᐦ ᒥᐧᔮᑭᒥᐱᔨᔨᐤ ᐅᒥᐦᒄ; ᐋᑳ ᒫᒃ ᐴᓃᒑ, ᓈᔥᑎᔨᒡ ᓂᒥ ᐧᐃᔮᔥ ᒋᑭ ᒌᐦ ᐧᐄᒋᐦᐄᑰ ᑯᑎᒋᔨᐤ ᒑᐧᑳᔨᐤ᙮ ᐊᑯᑖᐦ ᒫᒃ ᒑ ᒌᐦ ᐄᐢᐱᔨᐦᐅᑦ ᐊᓂᑖᐦ ᐱᑯᑎᐢᑭᒥᑳᐦᒡ ᒑ ᒌᐦ ᐃᐦᑖᑦ᙮ ᓈᐅᔥ ᒫᒃ ᒌᐦ ᐃᐦᑎᐤ ᐊᓂᔮ ᒨᔥ ᐋᐦ ᐅᒋᐧᑳᒋᒑᑦ, ᐋᐦ ᐱᐹᒥᐱᔨᑦ ᐊᓂᑖᐦ ᓂᑑᐦᐆᐢᒌᐦᒡ᙮ ᒌᐦ ᒥᐧᔮᔨᐦᑎᒼ᙮ ᐋᑯᑖᐦ ᐧᐋᔥ ᓈᔥᒡ ᒫᐅᒡ ᑳᐦ ᒥᐧᔮᔨᐦᑎᐦᒃ ᐋᐦ ᐄᐦᑖᑦ᙮

ᐊᓂᑖᐦ ᒫᒃ ᐧᐋᐧᓵᓂᐲ ᓂᑐᐦᑯᔨᓂᑭᒥᑯᐦᒡ ᒌ ᐃᐦᑖᔨᐤᐦ ᐊᓂᑖᐦ ᐋᐦ ᐅᐢᒋᓯᔨᒡᐦ ᐊᐧᐋᔨᐤᐦ ᐋᐦ ᐧᐄᒋᐦᐋᔨᒡᐦ ᑯᐃᐢᑯ ᒑ ᒌᐦ ᐄᔑ ᒦᒋᓯᔨᒡᐦ ᐊᐧᐋᔨᐤᐦ ᐋᔭᐧᐃᑯᓐᐦ ᒨᔥ ᑳ ᒌ ᓂᑎᐧᐋᐱᒫᑦ ᒑᒃ᙮ ᒌᐦ ᐧᐋᐧᐄᐦᑎᒫᑰ ᑖᓂᑖᐦ ᓈᐦᐋᐤ ᐋᔑᓈᑯᓂᔨᒡ ᐊᐧᐋᓐ ᓈᔥᒡ ᐋᐦ ᓈᑭᑎᐧᐋᔨᐦᑎᐦᒃ ᐋᔑ ᒦᒋᓯᑦ, ᑭᔮᐦ ᑖᓂᑖᐦ ᒑ ᒌᐦ ᐅᐦᒋ ᐧᐄᒋᐦᑖᑦ ᐊᐧᐋᓐ ᐋᑳ ᓈᔥᒡ ᒑ ᒌᐦ ᒫᑯᐦᐄᑯᑦ ᐋᐦ ᔔᑳᐅᐱᔨᑦ᙮ ᒌᐦ ᐧᐄᐦᑎᒫᑰ ᐊᓂᔮ ᒑᐧᑳᔨᐤ ᐋᐦ ᓈᔥᑎᔨᒡ ᐧᐄᒋᐦᐄᐧᐋᔨᒡ ᐋᐦ ᔔᑳᐅᐱᔨᓈᓂᐧᐃᐧᐃᔨᒡ (ᐲᐧᓵᔮᐦᑯᓈᐤᐦ, ᔔᑳᔨᐤ, ᑳᐲᔥᒑᐅᐱᔨᔑᔨᒡ,

ᐊᓂᑕ ᐊᓐ ᒉᐧᑳᒡ = ᓇᒧᐃ ᐅᐦᒋ ᐃᐦᑖᑯᓂᔮ ᑖᓂᑌ ᒉᒌ ᐅᐦᒋ ᐧᐄᒋᐦᐋᑲᓅᑦ᙮ ᒌ ᐃᐦᑑᑕᒼ ᒫᒃ ᐁᑳ ᒉᒌ ᐊᐃᐦᑖᑦ ᐊᓂᑌ ᐅᐧᐄᒉᐧᐋᑲᓐᐦ ᐁ ᐃᐦᑖᔨᒡ ᐊᓂᔮᐦ ᑮᐹ ᑲ ᐧᐄᐦᒋᐸᔨᐧᑖᐤ ᐧᐁᐢ ᓈᓂᑑ ᒦᓐ ᑳᐤ ᒋᐹ ᐧᐄᒋᒥᐦᓂᐦᐧᑫᒉᐤ᙮ ᐁᐅᒄ ᒥᒄ ᑳ ᒪᒉᒋᒥᓇᐦᒃ ᐊᓂᔮ ᑲ ᐃᔑ ᐊᔨᒥᐦᐄᑯᑦ ᓂᑐᐦᑯᐃᓐᐦ ᐁᑳ ᒉᒌ ᒥᓂᐦᐧᑫᑦ ᑲᔦ ᐁᑳ ᒉᒌ ᐅᑎᓇᐦ ᒪᒋᓂᑐᐦᑯᐃᓐᐦ, ᐅᔮ ᐃᔑ ᓇᓈᑲᑐᐧᐁᔨᐦᑕᐦᑫ ᒋᑲᒌ ᐃᔑᓈᑯᓂᔮ ᒉᒌ ᒥᔮᐸᔨᑦ ᐅᐲᒫᑎᓰᐧᐃᓂᐦᒡ ᐁᑳ ᑖᐱᔑᒫᑲᓅᑦ᙮ ᐁᑳ ᒫᒃ ᒉ ᐅᐦᒋ ᐴᓂᔨᐧᑫ, ᓇᒧᐃ ᒥᒍᓐ ᐅᐦᒋ ᐃᐦᑕᑯᓂᔮ ᑖᓐ ᒦᓐ ᒋᐹᒌ ᐃᔑ ᐧᐄᒋᐦᐋᑲᓅᑦ᙮ ᒌ ᐃᐦᑕᑯᓂᔮ ᑮᐹ ᐊᓂᑌ ᓅᐦᒋᒦᐦᒡ ᑖᓂᑌ ᒉᒌ ᓂᑑ ᐃᐦᑖᑦ᙮ ᑕᐦᐧᑖᐤ ᑳᐦ ᒨᔑᐦᑖᑦ ᐁᐧᐄ ᒥᓂᐦᐧᑫᑦ ᒌ ᓂᑑ ᐅᒋᐧᑳᒉᐤ, ᒫᒃ ᒌ ᓂᑑ ᐸᐹᒥᐸᔮ ᐅᑖᐹᓐ ᐁ ᐋᐸᒋᐦᑖᑦ ᒫᒃ ᓅᐦᒋᒦᐦᒡ ᒌ ᓂᑑ ᐃᐦᑖᐤ᙮ ᒋᓀᐅᔥ ᒫᒃ ᐁᐅᒄ ᑳ ᐃᐦᑎᑦ ᐁ ᓂᑑ ᐅᒋᐧᑳᒉᑦ ᒫᓐᐦ, ᐁ ᐸᐹᒥᐸᔨᑦ ᑲᔦ ᓅᐦᒋᒦᐦᒡ ᐁ ᓂᑑ ᐃᐦᑖᑦ᙮ ᒨᔥ ᐁᑯᓐ ᑳᐯᒋ ᐃᔑᓈᑯᓯᑦ ᐁ ᒥᔦᔨᐦᑕᐦᒃ ᐹ ᑮᐊᓂᑌ ᓅᐦᒋᒦᐦᒡ ᐁ ᐃᑖᑦ᙮

ᒌ ᓂᑐᐧᐋᐸᒉᐤ ᑲᔦ ᒫᓐ ᐊᓂᔮᐦ ᑳ ᐧᐋᐧᐄᒋᐦᐋᔨᒡ ᐊᐧᐁᔮᐦ ᒉᐃᔑ ᒥᔮᒦᒋᓯᔨᒡ ᐊᓂᑌ ᐧᐋᐢᐧᐊᓂᐲ ᓂᑐᐦᑯᐃᓂᑲᒥᑯᐦᒡ ᑳ ᐋᐸᑎᓯᔨᒡ᙮ ᐧᐁᒌᐦᒡ ᑳ ᐧᐋᐧᐄᐦᑕᒫᑯᑦ ᒉᐧᑳᔮᐦ ᒋᐹ ᒦᒎ ᑲᔦ ᑖᓐ ᐁ ᐃᔑ ᐋᐸᑎᓰᒪᑲᓂᔨᐧᑳᐤ ᐊᓂᑌ ᐲᐦᒌᔮ ᑲᔦ ᒌ ᐧᐄᐦᑕᒫᑰ ᒉᒄ ᒦᒋᒼᐦ ᒉ ᐧᐄᒋᐦᐄᑯᑦ ᐁ ᔒᐧᐋᑲᒥᐦᐧᑫᑦ᙮ ᐃᐦᑕᑯᓐᐦ ᒦᒋᒼ ᐁ ᐃᐦᑑᑖᒉᒪᑲᐦᐧᑳᐤ ᐁᑎᑑ ᒉᒌ ᐃᐢᐧᑲᐦᒋᐸᔨᔨᒡ ᐊᐧᐁᓐ ᐅᔔᑲᒼ ᒨᔭᒼ ᐲᐧᓴᐊᐦᑯᓈᐤ, ᐁ ᓰᑳᐅᐦᐧᑳᐤ ᒦᒋᒼᐦ, ᑳᐲᔥᑌᐅᐸᔨᐦᒡ, ᐸᐦᐧᑫᔑᑲᓂᐦᒡ ᐁᒌ ᐅᐦᒋ ᐅᔑᐦᑖᑲᓅᐦᒡ ᒦᒋᒼ ᑲ ᐅᔑᑲᓅᐦᐧᑳᐤ, ᐁᒄ ᐊᓂᔮ

il n’avait aucun groupe de soutien. Il dut même arrêter de fréquenter certains de ses amis les plus proches pendant un certain temps parce que, même si c’étaient des gens bien, quand il était avec eux, il avait envie de boire. Ce qu’il possédait c’était un savoir, le savoir que s’il arrêtait de boire et de se droguer, il avait une chance de mener une vie agréable, sans dialyse; s’il n’arrêtait pas, il n’avait aucune chance. Et il avait le bois. Chaque fois qu’il voulait boire, il allait à la pêche ou faire un tour en voiture, ou encore sur le territoire. Pendant longtemps, il sembla que Jack passait la plupart de son temps à pêcher, à conduire ou dans le bois. Cette partie n’était pas si mal. Le bois avait toujours été son endroit préféré.

group. In fact, he had to stop hanging out with some of his closest friends for a while because, even though they were good people, when he was with them he wanted to drink. What he had was the knowledge that if he quit drinking and quit drugs, he stood a chance at a good life without dialysis; if he didn’t quit, he had no chance at all. And he had the bush. Every time he wanted to drink, he went fishing, or for a drive, or out on the land. For a long time, it seemed that Jack spent most of his time fishing, driving, or out in the bush. That part wasn’t so bad. The bush had always been his favourite place to be.

Jack commença à parler avec la nouvelle nutritionniste qui travaillait à la clinique de Waswanipi. Elle lui expliqua ce qu’était un régime alimentaire sain et comment le diabète fonctionne dans le corps. Elle lui apprit aussi à gérer son diabète par l’alimentation. Certains aliments aggravaient la situation (pain, sucre, bière, pâte) et certains aliments l’aidaient (viandes traditionnelles, légumes). En fait, il apprit qu’il y avait beaucoup de choses

Jack began to speak with the new nutritionist who worked at the Waswanipi clinic. She explained to him what a healthy diet actually was and how diabetes works in the body, and she taught him ways to manage his diabetes with food. There were foods that made it worse (breads, sugars, beer, pastas) and foods that helped (traditional meats, vegetables). In fact, he learned, there were quite a few things he could have

ᐱᐦᐧᑳᔑᑭᓂᐦᒡ ᐋᐦ ᐅᐦᒋ ᐅᔑᐦᑳᑭᓂᐧᐃᐧᐃᔨᒡ ᒦᒋᒥᔨᐤ) ᑮᔮᐦ ᐊᓂᔮ ᓈᔥᒡ ᐧᐋᒋᐦᐄᑯᑦ ᐊᐧᐋᓐ (ᐄᔨᒦᒋᒥᔨᐤ, ᐊᔅᒌᐦᒡ ᐋᐦ ᓂᐦᑖᐅᒋᓂᔨᒡ ᒑᐧᑳᔨᐤ)᙮ ᐋᑯᑎᐦ ᑳᐦ ᐅᐦᒋ ᒋᔅᒑᔨᐦᑎᐦᒃ ᓂᔮᑭᓐᐦ ᑯᐃᔅᒄ ᒌᐦ ᐧᐄᐦᑎᒧᐧᐋᑭᓂᐧᐃᑦ ᑖᓐ ᐋᔑᓈᑯᓂᔨᒡ ᐊᓂᔮ ᑯᐃᔅᒄ ᐋᐦ ᐄᔑ ᒦᒋᓯᑦ ᐊᐧᐋᑉ ᐊᑐᒡ ᐧᐄ ᐧᔖᑳᐅᐱᔨᐤ᙮ ᑖᐹ ᒫᒃ ᐅᐦᒋ ᒋᔅᒑᔨᐦᑎᒻ ᐅᔮ᙮ ᐋᑦ ᑭᔨᐧᐸ ᑳᐦ ᒋᔅᒑᔨᐦᑎᒥᐧᑳ, ᑖᐹ ᓈᔥᒡ ᐅᐦᐦᒋ ᓈᓈᑭᒋᐦᑖᐤ᙮ ᓂᔮᔪ ᐲᓯᒻ ᒫᒃ ᑳ ᐄᔥᐱᔑ ᐴᓃᑦ ᐋᐦ ᒥᓂᐦᐧᑳᑦ ᑮᔮᐦ ᑯᐃᔅᒄ ᐋᐦ ᐄᔑ ᒦᒋᓯᑦ ᒦᓐ ᑳᐦ ᐄᔅᐱᔨᑦ ᒑᒃ ᐊᓂᑖᐦ ᐧᒫᓐᑎᓅᐧᔮᑦ ᐊᓂᔮᐦ ᓂᑐᐦᑯᔨᓂᑭᒥᑯᔨᐤ ᐊᓂᑖᐦ ᐋᐦ ᒦᔥᑯᑎᒧᐦᑖᑭᓂᐧᐃᐧᐃᔨᒡ ᒑᐧᑳᔨᐤ ᐊᐧᐋᓐ ᐲᐦᒡ ᐅᔮᐦᒡ ᐋᐦ ᐅᐦᒋ ᐱᒦᐦᑭᐧᐋᑭᓂᐧᐃᑦ᙮

ᓈᔥᒡ ᒥᒋᓐ ᐋᐦ ᒌᐦ ᓂᑑᑎᐹᔨᒫᑭᓂᐧᐃᑦ ᑮᔮᐦ ᒥᔥᑏᐦ ᐋᐦ ᒌᐦ ᑯᐧᑳᒋᒫᑭᓂᐧᐃᑦ ᒑᐧᑳᔨᐤ᙮ ᐊᓂᔮᐦ ᐋᐦ ᒦᔥᑯᑎᒧᐦᑖᑭᓂᐧᐃᐧᐃᔨᒡ ᐊᐧᐋᓐ ᒑᐧᑳᔨᐤ ᐅᔮᐦᒡ ᓈᔥᑖᐧᐹᐦ ᐋᔨᒥᓐ ᑮᔮᐦ ᐋᔪᐧᐃᒄ ᔮᔨᑖ ᐋᔑ ᓂᑎᐧᐋᔨᐦᑖᑯᓯᑦ ᐊᐧᐋᓐ ᒑ ᒥᔪᐋᐱᑎᓰᒥᑭᓂᔨᒡ ᐅᑖᐃᐦ ᒑ ᒑᐦ ᐧᔖᐳᔥᑭᐦᒡ ᐊᓂᔮ ᒫᒋᐧᔖᑭᓂᐧᐃᐧᐃᒑ᙮ ᑮᔮᐦ ᐋᐅᒄ ᐧᐋᐦ ᒑᔥᑎᓈᐦᐅᓈᓂᐧᐃᒡ ᐊᓐ ᐊᐧᐋᓐ ᒑ ᒥᔮᑭᓂᐧᐃᑦ ᔮᔨᑖ ᑯᐃᔅᒄ ᒑ ᓈᓈᑭᒋᐦᐄᓯᑦ᙮ ᒥᔑᐤ ᒫᒃ ᒦᓐ ᒥᓂᐦᐧᑳᒑ ᑮᔮᐦ ᐋᑳ ᑯᐃᔅᒄ ᐄᔑ ᒦᒋᓯᒑ ᓈᔥᑖᐧᐹᐦ ᐧᐄᐱᒡ ᓂᒥ ᒋᑭ ᐋᐱᑎᓰᒥᑭᔨᐤᐦ ᐊᓂᔮ ᑳ ᒥᔮᑭᓂᐧᐃᑦ᙮ ᑮᔮᐦ ᐋᐱᒥᔥᑖᑭᐦᐋᑭᓂᐅ ᐊᐧᐋᓐ ᓂᑐᐦᑯᔨᓐᐦ ᐊᓂᑎᐦ ᒑ ᒌᐦ ᐅᐦᒋ ᓂᐦᐄᔥᑳᑯᑦ ᐊᓂᔮ ᑳ ᒥᔮᑭᓂᐧᐃᑦ ᐅᔮᐦᒡ᙮ ᓂᒥᐧᐋᐧᐋᒡ ᐹᔨᐧᑲ ᒋᑭ ᒌᐦ ᐧᐃᓂᒋᔅᒋᓯᐤ ᐊᐧᐋᓐ ᒑ ᐅᑎᓂᐦᒃ ᐊᓂᔮᐦ ᓂᑐᐦᑯᔨᓐᐦ᙮ ᐊᓂᔮ ᒫᒃ ᑳ ᐄᔑ ᓈᓂᑑᒋᔅᒑᔨᐦᑖᑯᓯᑦ ᑮᔮᐦ ᑳ ᐄᔑ ᑯᐧᑳᒋᒫᑭᓂᐧᐃᑦ ᓈᔥᒡ ᓈᐅᔥ ᐋᐦ ᒌᐦ

ᒉᔫᔅᑳᒉᒪᑲᐦᐧᑳᐤ ᒎᔮᒻ ᐄᓂᒦᒋᒻ ᐁ ᐧᐄᔮᓰᐦᒡ, ᓂᐦᑖᐅᒋᐦᒋᑲᓐ ᒦᒋᒻ ᐊᓂᔫᐦ ᐁᑳ ᑳ ᔩᐧᐋᐧᑳᐤ᙮ ᐁᑯᑦ ᑳ ᐅᐦᒋ ᒋᔅᑫᔨᐦᑕᐦᒃ ᐁᒌ ᒥᔖᔨᑯᐸᓄ ᑖᓐ ᒋᐹᒌ ᐃᐦᑎᑯᐸᓄ ᒉᒌ ᐧᐄᒋᐦᑖᑦ ᐊᓂᔫ ᐅᑎᑖᔅᐱᓄᐧᐃᓐ᙮ ᓇᒧᐃ ᒫᒃ ᐅᐦᒋ ᒋᔅᑫᔨᐦᑕᒻ᙮ ᐋᑦ ᒌ ᒋᔅᑕᔨᐦᑕᐦᒃ ᓇᒧᐃ ᓈᓂᑑ ᒋᐹ ᐅᐦᒋ ᐋᐸᑌᔨᐦᑕᒻ᙮ ᐃᔅᑯᑕᒃ ᓂᔮᐃᓇ ᐲᓯᒻᐦ ᐁᑳ ᐅᐦᒋ ᒥᓂᐦᐧᑫᑦ ᑲᔦ ᐁᒌ ᒋᐦᒋᐸᔨᐦᑖᑦ ᑯᐃᔅᒄ ᐁ ᐃᔑ ᒦᒋᓯᑦ, ᐁᑯ ᑳ ᐃᔅᐸᔨᑦ ᒎᑖᔨᐦᒡ ᐊᓂᑌ ᒉ ᓂᑑ ᒋᔅᑫᔨᐦᑕᐦᒃ ᒉ ᐄᑖᑲᓅᐧᑫ ᒉᒋ ᒫᑎᐧᓵᑲᓅᐧᑫ᙮

ᒥᓯᐧᐁ ᒌᔑ ᓂᑑ ᒋᔅᑫᔨᒫᑲᓅ ᑲᔦ ᓇᓈᐦᑰ ᒌᔑ ᑲᐧᑫᒋᒫᑲᓅ᙮ ᐊᓂᔫ ᐁᐧᐄᔑ ᒫᒋᐧᔖᑲᓅᑦ ᐊᐧᐁᓐ ᓈᔅᒡ ᑖᐧᐯ ᔮᐧᑳᐤ ᐃᐦᑎᓈᓅ ᐁᒄ ᐅᑌᐦᐄ ᑲᔦ ᑳ ᓂᑑ ᒋᔅᑫᔨᐦᑖᑲᓄᔨᒡ ᑖᐧᐯ ᑫ ᓰᐦᒋᐸᐦᑲᐦᐄᑲᓄᔨᐧᑫ ᒫᒋᐧᔖᑲᓅᑌ᙮ ᒥᐦᑫᑑᒡ ᒫᒃ ᑯᑕᑲᒡ ᐊᐧᐁᓂᒌ ᐁ ᓂᑐᐧᐁᔨᑖᑯᓂᔨᒡ ᐅᔫ ᑫᒌᔑ ᒫᒋᐧᔖᑲᓅᐧᑖᐤ ᐁᑳ ᒫᒃ ᒌ ᐃᐦᑑᑐᐧᐋᑲᓅᐧᑖᐤ ᐁᐅᒄ ᒫᒃ ᐊᓂᔪ ᐧᐁᐦᒡ ᓈᔅᒡ ᓰᐦᒃ ᐳᑯᓭᔨᒧᐧᑖᐤ ᑫᒋ ᒥᔫᑲᓇᐧᐁᔨᒥᓯᑦ ᒎᒃ ᐃᔅᑯᑕᒃ ᒌ ᒪᓂᓯᑲᓄᔨᐧᑳᐧᐁᓐ ᐊᓂᔫᐦ ᐁᑳ ᑳ ᒥᐧᔮᔨᐧᑳᐤ ᐊᓂᑌ ᐲᐦᒋᔫ ᐁ ᐃᐦᑖᑦ ᒦᔅᑯᒡ ᐁ ᒥᐧᔮᔨᐧᑳᐤ ᑫᒋ ᐊᔮᑦ᙮ ᐃᔑᓈᑯᓯᑌ ᒦᓐ ᑳᐤ ᑫ ᒥᓂᐦᐧᑫᐧᑫ ᒎᔥ ᑲᔦ ᐁᑳ ᓇᓈᑲᒋᐦᑖᑌ ᐁ ᐃᔑ ᒦᒋᓯᑦ ᐧᐄᐸᒡ ᒋᑲᒌ ᓂᐲᒪᑲᓂᔫᐦ ᐊᓂᔫ ᑳ ᐋᐦᑖᒧᐦᑖᑲᓄᔨᐧᑳᐤ ᐊᓂᑕ ᐲᐦᒋᔫ ᐁ ᐃᐦᑖᑦ᙮ ᐊᐧᐁᓐ ᒫᒃ ᐅᔫ ᐁᒌᔑ ᒫᒋᐧᔖᑲᓅᑦ ᑫ ᐃᔥᐱᔥ ᐱᒫᑎᓰᐧᑫ ᒎᔥ ᒋᑲ ᐅᑎᓇᒻ ᓂᑐᐦᑯᐃᓐ ᑫᒌ ᐅᐦᒋ ᒥᔫᐸᔨᔨᒡ ᐊᓂᔫ ᑳ ᐅᔅᑳᔨᒡ ᐧᐃᔫᐦᒡ

qu'il aurait pu faire il y a longtemps pour aider à gérer sa maladie. Il ne les connaissait tout simplement pas. Ou s'il les avait sus, il ne les avait pas prises au sérieux. Cinq mois après son dernier verre et après avoir commencé à manger différemment, il se rendit en voiture à la clinique de transplantation de Montréal.

done a long time ago to help manage the disease. He just hadn't known about them. Or if he had known, he hadn't taken them seriously. Five months after his last drink and after starting to eat differently, he drove himself back down to the transplant clinic in Montréal.

Ils l'examinèrent attentivement et lui posèrent des questions. La transplantation d'organes est l'une des opérations les plus extrêmes qui puissent être pratiquées. Ils devaient donc s'assurer que son cœur était assez fort pour survivre à l'opération. Et comme il y a plus de gens qui ont besoin d'organes que de gens qui en reçoivent, ils devaient s'assurer que Jack respecterait les nouveaux organes. S'il reprenait une vie de boisson et d'alimentation malsaine, il épuiserait très vite les organes. Et toute personne ayant subi une transplantation doit prendre des pilules pour convaincre le système immunitaire d'accepter les nouveaux organes. Ces pilules ne peuvent être oubliées, pas même une seule fois.

They looked him over carefully and asked him questions. Organ transplant is one of the most extreme surgeries that can be done so they had to be sure that his heart was strong enough to survive the surgery. And there are more people who need organs than who ever receive them so they had to be sure that Jack would respect the new organs. If he went back to a life of drinking and of eating in unhealthy ways, he would burn out the organs very quickly. And anyone who has had a transplant has to take pills to convince the immune system to accept the new organs. Those pills can't be forgotten even once. Their list of questions and tests was long and intense. But, by the time Jack left the clinic, he

ᐱᒦᐦᑭᐧᐋᑭᓂᐧᐃᑦ᙮ ᒥᒄ ᒫᒃ ᑳ ᒌᔥᑐᑎᐧᐋᑭᓂᐧᐃᑦ ᒑᒃ, ᔖᔥ ᒌᐦ ᒥᓯᓂᐦᐧᐋᑭᓂᐆ ᐧᐄᔭ ᑭᔮᐦ ᒑ ᒌᐦ ᒥᔮᑭᓂᐧᐃᑦ ᐊᓂᑖᐦ ᐄᔑ ᓃᔥᑖᒥᐦᒡ ᓂᐦᐄᐱᔭᒑ ᐊᓂᔮ ᐋᔑ ᓂᑎᐧᐋᔭᐦᑎᐦᒃ᙮ ᐄᔅᑯᑎᒃ ᒫᒃ ᐴᓂᐱᒫᓯᔭᒋᐦᐋ ᐊᐧᐋᔭᐤᐦ ᐋᐦ ᒥᔪᓯᔭᒡᐦ ᐅᑐᑎᐦᑯᓯᔭᐤᐦ ᑭᔮᐦ ᒫᒃ ᐅᐲᔥᐲᔥᑭᔭᐤᐦ, ᐋᑯᑎᐦ ᒑ ᒋᐦ ᒥᔮᑭᓂᐧᐃᑦ ᐊᓂᔮ ᒑᐧᑳᔭᐤ ᓈᑎᐧᐋᔭᐦᑎᐦᒃ᙮

ᐋᐦᐧᒫᔮᐦ ᒫᒃ ᒌᐦ ᒥᔮᑭᓂᐧᐃᑦ ᐱᑎᒫ ᑎᔮᐱᔑᒫᑭᓂᐧᐃᑦ ᒥᑎᑑᓐ ᒑ ᒌᐦ ᒥᐧᔮᑭᒥᐱᔭᐦᑖᑭᓂᐧᐃᐧᐃᔭᒡ ᐅᒥᐦᒄ᙮ ᔖᔥ ᓂᒥ ᐄᔥᐱᔑᔭᔭᐤᐦ ᐧᐄᔭ ᐅᑐᑎᐦᑯᓯᐤᐦ ᑭᔮᐦ ᓂᒥ ᒌᐦ ᐧᐃᔮᐧᐄᔮᐳᑖᔭᐤ ᐊᓂᔮ ᐋᑳ ᒥᐧᔮᔭᒡ ᒑᐧᑳᔭᐤ ᐅᒥᐦᑯᐦᒡ, ᒥᒄ ᒫᒃ ᐋᔪᐧᐃᒄ ᓈᔥᒡ ᓈᑎᐧᐋᔭᐦᑖᑯᓂᔭᒡ ᒑ ᒌᐦ ᓂᔮᑭᒥᔭᒡ ᐅᒥᐦᒄ ᐅᐦᒋ ᐊᓂᔮ ᒑ ᐄᔥᐱᔥ ᐋᐦᐧᑳᒡ ᒫᒋᐧᔖᑭᓂᐧᐃᑦ᙮ ᓃᓚ ᐲᓯᒻᐦ ᐄᔥᐱᔥ ᒌᐦ ᐄᑐᐦᑖᐤ ᐊᓂᑖᐦ ᐧᒫᓐᑎᓈᐧᔮᑦ ᓂᑐᐦᑯᔭᓂᑭᒥᑯᐦᒡ ᒑ ᑖᐱᔑᒫᑭᓂᐧᐃᑦ ᓂᔥᐧᑖᐤ ᐹᔭᑯᑎᐧᐃᔥᑖᐤᐦ ᑭᔮᐦ ᐋᑯᑎᐦ ᒑ ᐋᐱᑦ ᓈᐧᐋᐤ ᐋᐦ ᒌᓂᐧᑳᓂᐦᑖᔭᒡᐦ ᐲᓯᒧᐦᑳᓐᐦ ᒫᐧᑳᒡ ᐋᐦ ᒥᐧᔮᑭᒥᐦᑖᑭᓂᐧᐃᐧᐃᔭᒡ ᐅᒥᐦᒄ᙮ ᐋᑯᑎᐦ ᒫᒃ ᒦᓐ ᒥᐦᒑᑐ ᑳᐦ ᓂᒋᔥᑭᐧᐋᑦ ᐄᔭᔭᐤᐦ ᐋᐦ ᐧᐄᐦ ᐊᔭᒥᐦᐋᔭᒡᐦ ᐊᐧᐋᔭᐤᐦ ᑭᔮᐦ ᒌᐦ ᒥᐧᔮᔭᐦᑎᒻ ᒑᒃ ᐅᔮ ᒑ ᒌᐦ ᐃᐦᑐᑎᐦᒃ᙮

ᐹᔭᐧᑳᐤ ᒫᒃ ᐋᐦ ᒌᔑᑳᔭᒡ, ᒌᐦ ᐹᐦᑎᒻ ᐋᐦ ᒌᐦ ᐴᓂᐱᒫᑎᓯᔭᒡᐦ ᐊᐧᐋᔭᐤᐦ ᑭᔮᐦ ᐋᐦ ᒌᐦ ᐃᐦᑎᑯᓂᔭᒡ ᐊᓂᔮ ᒑᐧᑳᔭᐤ ᒑ ᒌᐦ ᒥᔮᑭᓂᐧᐃᑦ

ᑳ ᐊᔮᑦ᙮ ᓇᒧᐃ ᒋᑲᒌ ᐃᐦᑑ ᐊᐧᐁᓐ ᐧᐋᒋ ᐯᔭᐧᑳᐤ ᑫᒌ ᐧᐊᓂᒋᔅᒋᓯᑦ ᑫᒌ ᐅᑎᓇᐦᒃ ᐅᓂᑐᐦᑯᐃᓂᒻᐦ᙮ ᒋᓀᐅᔥ ᒌ ᑕᓰᐦᑲᐧᐋᑲᓅ ᓇᓅᐦᑰ ᐁ ᐃᔑ ᑲᐧᑫᒋᒫᑲᓅᑦ ᒑᒃ ᑲᔦ ᓇᓅᐦᑰ ᐁᐃᔑ ᓂᑑ ᒋᔅᑫᔮᒫᑲᓅᑦ᙮ ᐃᔅᑯᑕᒃ ᒫᒃ ᑳ ᐧᐄᐧᐄᑦ ᐊᓂᑕ ᓵᔅ ᒌ ᒪᓯᓇᐦᐧᐋᑲᓅ ᑫ ᒪᒋᐧᓵᑲᓅᑦ, ᓃᓚ ᑫᐧᑳᔫ ᐲᐦᒋᔪ ᐁ ᐃᐦᑖᑦ ᑫ ᒪᓂᔑᑲᓄᔭᐧᑳᐤ ᐁᒄ ᑯᑕᒃ ᑫ ᒋᑲᒧᐦᑖᑲᓄᔭᐧᑳᐤ ᑫ ᒦᔅᑯᒋᔅᑳᑫᒪᑲᓂᔭᐧᑳᐤ᙮ ᐹᑎᔅ ᑮᐹ ᒋᐹ ᐊᓚᐧᐋᐸᐦᑕᒻ ᑫᒌ ᓂᐱᔭᒡ ᐊᐧᐁᔫ ᐊᓂᑕ ᐧᐃᔪᐧᐃᔭᐦᒡ ᑫ ᐅᐦᒋ ᒪᓂᓯᑲᓄᔭᐧᑳᐤ ᐊᓂᔫᐦ ᑫᐧᑳᔫᐦ ᐧᐄᔭ ᓀᑐᐧᐁᔭᐦᑕᐦᒃ᙮

ᑫᐧᑳᒡ ᒫᒃ ᐁ ᐊᓚᐧᐋᐱᑦ, ᒌ ᑖᐱᔑᒫᑲᓅ ᐱᑕᒫ᙮ ᓵᔅ ᓇᒧᐃ ᐅᐦᒋ ᓵᐱᓯᔫᐦ ᐅᑌᐦᑕᑯᓯᔫᐦ ᑫᒌ ᑯᐃᐧᑳᓯᑯᐦᑖᔭᒡ ᐱᐦᒋᐳᐧᐋᐳᔫ ᐅᒥᐦᑯᐦᒡ ᐁᒄ ᒫᒃ ᑳ ᑖᐱᔑᒫᑲᓅᑦ ᐧᐁᔅ ᐁᐅᒄ ᐁ ᐄᑖᐸᑕᐦᒡ ᐁ ᑖᐱᔑᒫᑲᓅᑦ ᐊᐧᐁᓐ, ᐸᔦᐦᒋᐦᑖᑲᓅᔫ ᐅᒥᐦᒄ᙮ ᒌ ᓂᑐᐧᐁᔭᐦᑖᑲᓅᔫ ᑫᒌ ᒥᐧᔮᑲᒥᔭᒡ ᐅᒥᐦᒄ ᑲᔦ ᐅᑌᐦᐄ ᑫᒌ ᓰᐦᒋᓰᒪᑲᓂᔭᒡ ᑫᒌ ᔖᐳᔥᑲᐦᒃ ᐊᓂᔫ ᓈᔅᒡ ᔮᐧᑳᐤ ᐁ ᐃᐦᑑᑕᐧᐋᑲᓅᑦ ᐊᐧᐁᓐ ᐁ ᒫᒋᐧᔖᑲᓅᑦ᙮ ᐁᒄ ᓃᓚ ᐲᓯᒻ ᐃᔥᐱᔥ, ᒨᓕᔮᐦᒡ ᑳ ᓂᑑ ᐃᐦᑖᑦ ᓂᔥᐧᑖᐤ ᐯᔭᒄ ᑑᔥᑌᐤ ᑲᒌ ᑖᐱᔑᒫᑲᓅᑦ ᓀᐤ ᑎᐸᐦᐄᑲᓐᐦ ᐁᒌ ᐃᔥᐱᔥ ᐃᑕᐱᑦ ᒫᓐᐦ ᐁ ᐸᔦᐦᒋᐦᑖᑫᒪᑲᓄᔭᒡ ᐅᒥᐦᒄ᙮ ᐁᒄ ᑮᐹ ᒦᓐ ᑳ ᓇᒋᔥᑯᐧᐋᑦ ᐄᓅᐦ ᐁ ᓂᑐᐧᐁᔭᒫᔭᒡ ᑯᑕᒃ ᐄᓅᐦ ᑫᒌ ᐊᔭᒥᐦᐄᑯᐧᑖᐤ ᒌ ᒥᔦᔭᐦᑕᒻ ᒫᒃ ᒑᒃ ᐁ ᐊᔭᒥᐦᐋᑦ ᒫᓐ᙮

ᐯᔭᐧᑳᐤ ᒫᒃ ᐁ ᒌᔑᑳᔭᒡ ᒌ ᐯᐦᑕᒻ ᐁᒌ ᐴᓂᐱᒫᑎᓯᔭᒡ ᐊᐧᐁᔫ ᐁ ᐊᐧᐋᔒᐧᐃᔭᒡ ᐁᒄ ᑮᐹ ᑳ ᐃᐦᑕᑯᓂᔭᐧᑳᐤ ᐊᓂᔫᐦ ᑖᓐ ᑳ

Leur liste de questions et de tests était longue et intense. Toutefois, lorsque Jack quitta la clinique, il était sur une liste pour recevoir de nouveaux organes. Si une personne ayant des organes sains et des tissus correspondants mourait, il pourrait recevoir leurs organes.

was on a list for new organs. If someone with healthy organs and matching tissues died, he could receive their organs.

Entretemps, les médecins le mirent sous dialyse temporaire. Ses propres reins ne pouvaient plus éliminer toutes les toxines qu'ils étaient censés éliminer, mais son sang devait être exempt de toxines pour qu'il puisse survivre une opération aussi drastique. Pendant deux mois, il se rendit à la clinique de dialyse de Montréal trois fois par semaine et y restait assis pendant quatre heures alors que la grosse machine à dialyse nettoyait son sang. Là encore, il rencontra de nombreux Cris qui avaient besoin de quelqu'un à qui parler et Jack était heureux de le faire.

In the meantime, the doctors put him on temporary dialysis. His own kidneys could no longer flush out all the toxins they were supposed to flush out, but his blood had to be free of toxins if he was to live through such a rigorous surgery. For two months, he went into the Montréal dialysis clinic three times a week and sat there for four hours as the big dialysis machine cleaned his blood. Again, he met many Cree people there who needed someone to talk to and Jack was happy to oblige.

Un jour, il apprit que quelqu'un était mort prématurément et que des organes étaient devenus disponibles pour lui.

One day, he heard that someone had died too soon and organs had become available for him. But for some reason

ᐋᐦ ᓂᐦᐄᔥᑳᑯᑦ᙮ ᒥᒄ ᒫᒃ ᐊᓂᔮ ᑳᔑᑳᔭᒡ ᒑᒃ ᒌᐦ ᑭᒋᔅᓰ ᐋᑯᐦ ᓂᒥ ᐅᐦᒋ ᒌᐦ ᒫᒋᐧᔖᑭᓂᐆ᙮ ᑯᑎᒃᐦ ᐊᐧᐋᔭᐤᐦ ᑳᐦ ᒥᔮᑭᓂᐧᐃᐧᐃᔭᒡᐦ ᑳᐦ ᒥᓯᓈᓯᔭᒡᐦ ᐊᓂᔮ ᒑ ᒥᔮᑭᓂᐧᐃᑯᐱᓈ᙮ ᓂᒧᐃ ᒫᒃ ᓈᔥᒡ ᓈᐅᔥ ᐧᒫᐦᒡ ᒌᐦ ᐧᐄ ᐄᔅᐱᐦᔫᐤ ᐊᓂᑖᐦ ᐧᐋᐧᔖᓂᐲᐦᒡ ᐋᐦ ᐧᐄᐦ ᓂᑑᑭᐱᓯᑦ ᒦᓐ ᑯᑎᒃᐦ ᐊᐧᐋᔭᐤᐦ ᑳᐦ ᐴᓂᐱᒫᑎᓯᔭᒡᐦ᙮ ᐋᑯᑎᐦ ᐊᓂᑎᐦ ᐧᒫᓐᑎᓅᐧᔮᑦ ᑲ ᐃᐦᑖᑦ ᒑᒃ, ᐊᓂᔮ ᒫᒃ ᑳᔑᑳᔭᒡ ᐋᑯᑎᐦ ᑲ ᒥᔮᑭᓂᐧᐃᑦ ᑯᑎᒃᐦ ᐅᑐᑎᐦᑯᓰᐦ ᑭᔮᐦ ᐅᐲᔥᐲᔥᒃᐦ᙮

ᐅᑎᐦ ᒫᒃ ᒥᓯᓂᐦᐄᑭᓐᐦᒡ ᑖᐹᒋᒫᑭᓂᐧᐃᑦ ᐊᐧᐋᓐ ᐋᐅᒄ ᒑᒃ ᐧᔖᔥ ᓂᒥ ᐊᔫᐤ ᐋᐦ ᐧᔖᑳᐅᐱᔭᓈᓂᐧᐃᐧᐃᔭᒡ᙮ ᐋᔪᐧᐃᒄ ᐋᑯᐦ ᐊᓂᔮ ᐋᐦ ᐅᔅᒋᓯᔭᒡᐦ ᐅᐲᔥᐲᔥᒃ, ᑭᔮᐦ ᐋᐦ ᓂᐦᐄᔥᑳᑯᑦ ᐊᓂᑎᐦ ᐧᐋᔥᑖᒑᐳᐃᔭᔭᒡ ᐄᓐᓯᓚᓐ, ᐧᔖᔥ ᒦᓂᐧᐊᑎᔫᐤ᙮ ᒥᓯᐧᐋ ᐄᔑ ᒥᔦᐱᔭᔭᐤ ᐊᓂᔮ ᑳ ᒥᔮᑭᓂᐧᐃᑦ ᐋᐦ ᐅᔅᒋᓯᔭᒡ ᐅᐲᔥᐲᔥᒃᐦ ᑭᔮᐦ ᐊᓂᔮᐦ ᐅᑐᑎᐦᑯᓯᐤᐦ᙮ ᐊᓂᔮᐦ ᒫᒃ ᐋᐦ ᐄᔑ ᒥᔮᑭᓂᐧᐃᑦ ᐊᐧᐋᓐ ᓈᔥᑖᐧᐹᐦ ᓂᑎᐧᐋᔭᐦᑖᑯᓂᔭᐤ ᓈᔥᒡ ᒐ ᐧᐄᐦ ᓈᑭᑎᐧᐋᔭᒦᓯᑦ᙮ ᐋᑦ ᐧᔖᔥ ᐋᑳ ᐧᔖᑳᐅᐱᔭᑦ, ᓈᔥᑖᐧᐹᐦ ᑯᐃᔅᒄ ᐧᐄᐦ ᐄᔑ ᑭᓂᐧᐋᔭᒦᓰ, ᐊᓂᔮᐦ ᑳ ᐧᐄᐦ ᐄᔑ ᒥᔦᑭᓂᐧᐋᔭᒦᓯᑦ ᐊᓂᑖᐦ ᐄᔑ ᐅᑖᐦᒡ᙮ ᓂᒥ ᓈᔥᒡ ᐧᐄᐦ ᒦᒋᐤ ᐊᓂᔮ ᒦᒋᒥᔭᐤ ᐋᐦ ᒌᐦᐱᐦᑭᓯᑭᓂᐧᐃᐧᐃᔭᒡ, ᐧᐄᔭ ᐱᒥᓂᐆᑏᓰ (ᐅᔒ ᐧᐃᔮᐊᓯᔭᐤ ᑭᔮᐦ ᐊᓂᔮ ᐊᔅᒡᒌᐦᒡ ᐋᐦ ᓂᐦᑖᐅᒋᓂᔭᒡ ᒑᐧᑳᔭᐤ ᑭᔮᐦ ᐊᐱᔒᔥ ᐱᐦᐧᑳᔑᑭᓂᐦᒡ ᐋᐦ ᐅᐦᒋ ᐅᔑᐦᑖᑭᓂᐧᐃᐧᐃᔭᒡ ᒑᐧᑳᔭᐤ ᑭᔮᐦ ᒫᒃ ᐱᑖᑎᔅᐦ), ᑭᔮᐦ ᐧᔖᔥ ᓂᒥ ᒥᓂᐦᐧᑳᐤ ᒐ ᒌᐦ ᒥᔦᐦᑭᓯᑦ ᑭᔮᐦ ᓈᔥᑎᔭᒡ ᓂᒥ ᐱᒫᔭᐦᑎᒻ ᒥᒋᓂᑐᐦᑯᔭᓐᐦ᙮ ᐊᓂᑖᐦ ᒫᒃ

ᐃᔑ ᓂᑐᐧᐁᔭᐦᑕᐦᒃ ᐲᐦᒋᔫ᙮ ᐊᓂᔫ ᒫᒃ ᑳ ᒌᔑᑳᔭᒡ ᒉᐧᑳᒡ ᒌ ᐋᐦᑯᔥᑎᐧᑳᓃᐤ ᒑᒃ ᐁᒄ ᑳ ᓇᑳᐦᐄᑲᓅᔭᒡ ᐊᓂᔫ ᒋᐸ ᒫᒋᐧᔖᑲᓅ᙮ ᑯᑕᒃ ᐊᐧᐁᓐ ᐁᒌ ᒪᓯᓈᓯᑦ ᑫ ᒫᒋᐧᔖᑲᓅᑦ ᐁᐅᒄ ᑳ ᒥᔮᑲᓅᑦ ᐊᓂᔫ ᐧᐄᔭ ᒑᒃ ᒋᐸ ᐋᔮᐤ᙮ ᓇᒧᐃ ᒫᒃ ᒋᓀᐅᔥ ᒧᐧᐁᐦᒡ ᑫ ᐴᔑᑦ ᑳᐱᒥᐦᔮᒪᑲᓂᔭᒡ ᑫ ᒌᐧᐁᐦᐋᑦ ᑫ ᓂᑑ ᒌᐅᑌᑦ ᐧᐋᔅᐧᐋᓂᐲᐦᒡ ᑯᑕᒃ ᒦᓐ ᐊᐧᐁᓐ ᐁ ᐊᐧᐋᔒᐅᑦ ᒌ ᐴᓂᐱᑎᔫᐤ᙮ ᐁᑯᑌ ᒦᓐ ᑳ ᐃᐦᑖᑦ ᒧᑕᔮᐦᒡ ᑳ ᒫᒋᐧᔖᑲᓅᑦ ᐊᓂᔫ ᐊᔅᒌᐤ ᐊᒋᐦᒑᓯᓂᔫ 2012 ᑳ ᐃᒋᔥᑌᔭᒡ ᐁᑯᑦ ᑳ ᐅᔅᒋᓯᔭᒡ ᐅᑌᐦᑕᑯᓲᐦ ᑲᔦ ᐅᐦᐹᐱᑯᓲᒻ᙮

ᐁᐅᑰ ᒑᒃ ᐯᔭᒄ ᐊᐧᐁᓐ ᐅᑕ ᐆ ᒪᓯᓇᐦᐄᑲᓐ ᐁ ᐃᐦᑕᑯᓂᔭᒡ ᐅᑎᐹᒋᒧᐧᐃᓐ ᐯᔭᐧᑳᐤ ᐁᒌ ᓲᐧᐋᑲᒥᐦᐧᑫᑦ ᐁᑳ ᒫᒃ ᔖᔅ ᓲᐧᐋᑲᒥᐦᐧᑫᑦ᙮ ᐅᔅᑳᔫ ᐅᐦᐹᐱᑯᓲᒻ, ᒥᔫᐸᔭᓂᔫ, ᐁᐅᒄ ᒫᒃ ᐧᐁᐦᒋ ᒥᐧᔫᔭᒡ ᐅᓲᑳᒻ ᔖᔅ ᓇᒧᐃ ᐃᐦᑕᑯᓂᔫ ᐊᓂᔫ ᑲ ᐄᑖᔅᐱᓅᑦ ᐁᒌ ᓲᐧᐋᑲᒥᐦᐧᑫᐅᑦ᙮ ᒥᔅᑕᒥᔫᐸᔭᓂᔫ ᐊᓂᔫ ᑳ ᐅᔅᑳᔭᒡ ᐅᐦᐹᐱᑯᓲᒻ ᑲᔦ ᐊᓂᔫᐦ ᐅᑌᐦᑕᑯᓲ ᒥᔫᐸᔫᐦ᙮ ᐊᐧᐁᓐ ᐁ ᐅᔅᑳᔭᐧᑳᐤ ᐅᑫᐧᑳᓂᒻᐦ ᐲᐦᒋᔫ ᓂᑐᐧᐁᔭᐦᑖᑯᓲ ᔮᐧᑳᐤ ᑫᒌᔑ ᑲᓇᐧᐁᔭᒥᓯᑦ ᒋᓯᓄ ᑫᒌ ᒥᐧᔮᔭᐧᑳᐤ ᐊᓂᔫᐦ ᑳ ᒥᔮᑲᓅᑦ᙮ ᐋᑦ ᔖᔅ ᐁᑳ ᓲᐧᐋᑲᒥᐦᐧᑫᑦ ᒫᒃ, ᓄᐧᐊᒡ ᔮᐧᑳᐤ ᐃᔑ ᓇᓈᑲᑐᐧᐁᔭᒥᓰ ᐁᒄ᙮ ᓇᒧᐃ ᒦᒎ ᒦᒋᒥᔫ ᐁᑳ ᒥᔫᔅᑳᑫᒪᑲᓂᔭᒡ, ᐱᒥᓅᑎᓰ ᐅᔒᐦ ᐧᐃᔮᓯᔫ ᐁ ᒦᒋᑦ ᑲᔦ ᒫᒃ ᒦᒋᒻᐦ ᐁᒌ ᓂᐦᑖᐅᒋᐦᑖᑲᓅᔭᐧᑳᐤ ᒥᒄ ᐊᐱᔒᔥ ᒦᒎ ᐸᐦᐧᑫᔑᑲᓂᐦᒡ ᐁᒌ ᐅᐦᒋ ᐅᔑᐦᑖᑲᓅᔭᒡ ᒦᒋᒥᔫ ᑲᔦ ᓇᒧᐃ ᐃᔥᐱᔥ ᒦᒎ ᐸᑌᑎᔅ, ᓇᒧᐃ ᑲᔦ ᔖᔅ ᒥᓂᐦᐧᑫᐤ ᐃᔅᑯᑌᐧᐋᐳᔫ ᑲᔦ ᓇᒧᐃ ᐱᔅᑳᑕᒻ ᒪᒋᓂᑐᐦᑯᐃᓐᐦ ᐋᑦ ᒥᒄ ᐊᐱᔒᔥ ᑫᒌ ᐋᐸᒋᐦᑖᑦ᙮ ᓅᐦᒋᒦᐦᒡ ᒨᔥ ᒌ ᒥᔦᔭᐦᑕᒻ ᐁ ᐃᐦᑖᑦ ᐁᑯᑌ ᒫᒃ ᐅᔒ ᐁ ᐊᐃᐦᑖᑦ᙮

Toutefois, pour une raison quelconque, Jack avait de la fièvre ce jour-là et son opération dut être annulée. Les organes allèrent à quelqu'un d'autre sur la liste. Peu de temps après, Jack était sur le point de prendre un avion pour Waswanipi pour une visite, quand une autre personne mourut prématurément. Jack resta à Montréal et, ce jour-là, en 2012, il reçut un nouveau rein et un nouveau pancréas.

Jack est la seule personne dans ce livre qui était diabétique mais ne l'est plus désormais. Parce qu'il a un nouveau pancréas et parce que son corps accepte l'insuline que celui-ci produit, il est désormais guéri de la maladie. Son nouveau pancréas fonctionne à merveille et son nouveau rein se porte bien. Toutefois, les organes transplantés doivent être traités avec beaucoup de précaution. Même s'il n'est plus diabétique, il est plus vigilant que jamais quand il s'agit de sa santé. Il évite le *fast-food*, il cuisine ses propres repas (principalement de la viande et des légumes avec un peu de pâtes ou de pommes de terre), et il ne boit pas ni ne se drogue, pas même un peu. Comme le bois est l'endroit où il s'est toujours senti en meilleure santé, il passe le plus de temps possible sur

Jack had a fever that day and his surgery had to be cancelled. The organs went to someone else on the list. Not too long after that, Jack was about to catch a plane to Waswanipi for a visit when someone else died too soon. Jack stayed in Montréal and, on that day in 2012, he received a new kidney and a new pancreas.

Jack is the one person in this book who once had diabetes but no longer does. Because he has a new pancreas, and because his body accepts the insulin it creates, he is actually cured of the disease. His new pancreas works beautifully, and his new kidney feels fine. But transplanted organs have to be handled very carefully. Even though he no longer has diabetes, he is more vigilant about health than he ever was before. He avoids fast food, he cooks his own meals (mostly meat and vegetables with a little bit of pasta or potatoes), and he doesn't drink or do drugs even a little bit. Since the bush is where he has always felt healthiest, he spends as much time on the land as he can. He teaches his son the traditional ways of the land so that his son knows that even a robot leg and transplanted organs can't stop you from

ᓂᑑᐦᐆᔅᑏᐦᒡ ᐋᐦ ᐄᐦᑖᑦ ᐋᑯᑖᐦ ᒨᔥ ᑳ
ᐄᐦᑎᒥᒋᐦᐅᑦ ᓈᔥᒡ ᐋᐦ ᒥᔪᐱᒫᑎᓰᑦ, ᐋᑯᑖᐦ ᒫᒃ
ᒥᒄ ᐋᔥᐱᔥ ᒌᐦ ᐃᐦᑐᑎᐦᒃ ᐋᐦ ᐃᐦᑖᑦ ᐊᓂᑖᐦ᙮
ᒋᔅᑯᑎᒧᐧᐋᐤ ᐅᑯᓯᔅᐦ ᐊᓂᔮᐦ ᑭᔮᐦ ᐧᐄᔨ ᑳ
ᐄᔑ ᒋᔅᑯᑎᒧᐧᐋᑭᓂᐧᐃᑦ ᐄᔨᔨᐅᐃᔨᐦᑎᐧᐃᓂᔨᐤ
ᑭᔮᐦ ᐋᑯᑎᐦ ᐧᐋᐦᒋ ᒋᔅᒑᔨᐦᑎᒥᔨᒡᐦ ᐋᑦ
ᒥᔅᑳᑎᐦᑳᓂᔨᐤ ᐃᔮᔨᒡᐦ ᐊᐧᐋᔨᐤᐦ ᑭᔮᐦ ᐋᐦ
ᒌᐦ ᒦᔥᑯᑎᒧᐦᒑᑭᓂᐧᐃᐧᐃᔨᒡ ᒑᐧᑳᔨᐤ ᐅᔮᔨᐦᒡ
ᐊᔮᐱᒡ ᒋᑭ ᒌᐦ ᐃᐦᑖᐤ ᐊᐧᐋᓐ ᐊᓂᑖᐦ
ᓂᑑᐦᐆᔅᑏᐦ ᐧᐄᐦ ᐃᐦᑖᒐ, ᓂᒧᐃ ᒑᐧᑳᔨᐤ ᒋᑭ
ᒌᐦ ᒋᐱᐦᒋᐦᐄᑰ᙮ ᓂᑑᐦᐆ ᑭᔮᐦ ᓂᐱᐦᐋᐤ ᒨᔅᐦ
ᑭᔮᐦ ᑯᑎᒋᔨᐤ ᒦᒋᒥᔨᐤ ᑭᔮᐦ ᑎᑭᓯᒻ᙮ ᔒᔒᐧᐄᐤ
ᑭᔮᐦ ᐊᔮᔥᐱᔒᒡᐦ᙮ ᐋᐦᑯᓯᐤ ᓂᔮᓂᑰᓐᐦ ᐅᓇᑭᓐ
ᐅᐦᒋ ᐊᓂᔮ ᐋᐦ ᒥᔥᑖᐱᑎᓰᑦ ᐋᐦ ᐅᔅᑳᑎᐦᑳᓂᑦ
ᑭᔮᐦ ᐹᒋᐱᔨᐤ ᐅᐦᒋ ᐊᓂᔮ ᐋᐦ ᔒᔒᐧᐄᑦ, ᒥᒄ
ᒫᒃ ᓂᑎᐧᐋᔨᐦᑖᑯᓂᔨᐤ ᐊᐧᐋᓐ ᒑ ᔒᔒᐧᐄᑦ
ᐧᐄᐦ ᒥᔪᐱᒫᑎᓰᒐ, ᐋᑯᑖᐦ ᒫᒃ ᐋᐦᑎᐦᒃ ᑭᔮᐦ
ᒑᒃ᙮ ᐊᓂᑖᐦ ᒫᒃ ᓈᔥᒡ ᒥᔮᑯᐦᐄᑯᒡ ᒑᐧᑳᔨᐤ ᒑᒃ
ᐅᐱᒫᑎᓰᐧᐃᓂᐦᒡ, ᐋᔨᒥᐦᐋᑦ ᒋᔒᔨᔨᐤᐦ, ᐋᑯᐦ
ᒥᔮᑯᐦᐄᑯᒡᐦ ᒑᐧᑳᔨᐤ ᐅᐦᒋ ᐅᑖᐱᔅᑎᓰᐧᐃᓐ
ᐃᐦᑖᔨᐤᐦ ᐊᐧᐋᔨᐤᐦ ᒑ ᐧᐄᒋᐦᐄᑯᑦ ᐋᑯᐦ ᒦᔥᑯᒡ
ᓂᒥ ᑭᓂᐧᐋᔨᐦᑎᒫᓯᒌ ᐊᓂᑖᐦ ᐲᐦᒋᔨᐤ ᑭᔮᐦ
ᐅᔥᑎᐧᑳᓂᐦᒡ ᐧᐄᐱᒡ ᐋᐦ ᐧᐄᒋᐦᐄᓯᑦ᙮

ᓂᔮᓂᑰᓐᐦ ᒋᔅᒋᓰᑎᑎᒻ ᐊᓂᔮ ᒑᐧᑳᔨᐤ ᑳ
ᐹᐦᑎᐦᒃ ᐋᑳ ᑖᐧᐹᒥᑭᓂᔨᒡ᙮ ᓂᐧᐃᒡ ᒥᔥᑎᐦᐦ
ᒌᐦ ᐹᑎᒻ ᑳ ᐃᔥᐱᔑ ᐹᒋ ᐱᒫᑎᓰᑦ᙮ ᐧᑳᐧᔒᒡ
ᒫᒃ ᒌᐦ ᐄᔑᓈᑯᓂᔨᒡ ᑯᐃᔅᒄ ᒌᐦ ᐄᔑ
ᐧᐄᐦᑎᒧᐧᐋᑭᓂᐧᐃᑦ ᒫᐧᑳᒡ ᑳ ᐊᐧᐋᔑᔒᐧᐃᑦ,
ᐊᑐᒡ ᓈᓂᑎᐤ ᒋᐱᐦᒌ ᐄᔥᐱᔑ ᒫᑯᐦᐄᑰ ᐋᐦ
ᔖᑳᐅᐱᔨᑦ ᑭᔮᐦ ᐧᑳᐧᔒᓐ ᐋᔥᒄ ᒋᐱᐦᒌ ᐊᔮᐤ
ᐧᐄᔨ ᐊᓂᔮ ᑎᐲᔨᐧᐋ ᐅᔅᑳᑦ, ᐅᑐᑎᐦᑯᓯᐤᐦ
ᑭᔮᐦ ᒫᒃ ᐅᐲᔥᐲᔥᑲᐦ᙮ ᓂᔮᓂᑰᓐᐦ ᒫᒃ ᐋᔥᒄ

ᒋᔅᑯᑕᒧᐧᐁᐤ ᐅᑯᔅ ᐄᓅ ᐃᐦᑐᐧᐃᓂᔫ ᒉᒌ
ᒋᔅᒉᔨᐦᑕᒥᔨᒡ ᐋᑦ ᐁ ᓇᐸᑌᑳᑌᑦ ᐊᐧᐁᓐ ᑲᔦ
ᐁᒌ ᐅᔅᒋᐦᑖᑲᓈᔨᒡ ᒉᐧᑳᔫ ᐲᐦᒋᔫ ᐧᐃᔩᐦᒡ ᐁᑳ
ᒉ ᐅᐦᒋ ᓇᑳᐦᐆᑯᑦ ᒉᐧᑳᔫ ᐁᐧᐄ ᐃᐦᑑᑕᐦᒃ
ᐊᓂᑌᐦ ᓅᐦᒋᒦᐦᒡ ᐁ ᐃᐦᑖᑦ᙮ ᓂᑑᐦᐆ ᑲᔦ, ᐁ
ᐊᐱᔒᔑᔨᒡ ᒉᐧᑳᔫ ᓂᐸᐦᑖᐤ ᐁᒄ ᒉ ᑕᑲᔑᒃ
ᐊᓂᔫ ᐅᓂᐱᐦᑖᒉᐧᐃᓐ᙮ ᔖᔖᐧᐃᔫ ᐁ ᐃᔅᐱᔩᒡ
ᒫᓐᐦ᙮ ᓂᔮᓂᑯᑌᐦᒡ ᐅᔅᐱᔅᑯᓐ ᒨᔑᐦᑖᐤ ᐧᐁᔅ
ᒥᔅᑖᐸᑎᔩᒪᑲᓂᔫ ᐊᓂᔫ ᐅᔅᑳᑦ ᑳ ᒋᒫᔨᒡ ᐁ
ᒋᒋᔅᑲᐦᒃ ᒥᔅᑳᑎᐦᑳᓂᔫ, ᐁᒄ ᐊᓂᔫ ᑯᑕᒋᔫ
ᑳ ᒥᐧᔮᔨᒡ ᐅᔅᑳᑦ ᐹᒋᐸᔨᓂᔫ ᒫᓐ ᓰᐦᒃ
ᔮᐸᒋᐦᑖᒡ ᒥᒄ ᒫᒃ ᓂᑐᐧᐁᔨᐦᑖᑯᓂᔫ ᒨᔥ ᒉᒌ
ᔖᔖᐧᐃᔨᑦ ᒉᒌ ᒥᔫᐸᔨᑦ ᐧᐃᔩᐦᒡ᙮ ᐃᔅᑯᑕᒃ
ᒣᑯᔥᑳᑌᔨᐦᑕᒥᐦᐄᑯᑦ ᒉᐧᑳᔫ ᐅᐱᒫᑎᓰᐧᐃᓂᐦᒡ
ᒋᒋᐃᓅᐦ ᓂᑐᐧᐋᐸᒣᐤ ᐁᒄ ᐊᓂᑌ ᐁ ᐋᐸᑎᓯᑦ
ᐁ ᐅᔥᑕᐧᐁᔨᐦᑕᒥᐦᐄᑯᑦ ᒉᐧᑳᔫ ᐃᐦᑖᔫ ᐊᐧᐁᔫ
ᐊᓂᑌ ᐁ ᐊᔭᒥᐦᐋᑦ ᐁ ᐧᐄᐦᑕᒧᐧᐋᑦ ᑖᓐ ᐁ
ᐃᔅᐸᔨᑦ ᐁᒄ ᒫᒃ ᓇᒧᐃ ᓈᔅᒡ ᒫᐦᑕᑯᔅᑳᑰ
ᒥᒋᐦᐱᓐ ᑳ ᐧᐄᐧᐄᐸᔨᐦᑖᑦ ᑖᓐ ᐁ ᐃᑕᒪᐦᒋᐦᐅᑦ᙮

ᓂᔮᓂᑯᑌᐦᒡ ᑲᔦ ᓂᑕᒧᒄ ᒉᐧᑳᔫᐦ
ᒫᒥᑐᓀᔨᐦᑕᒥᐦᐄᑰ᙮ ᒥᔅᑕᐦᐄ ᒉᐧᑳᔫ ᒌ ᐯᐦᑕᒻ
ᒥᐦᒉᑐ ᐱᐳᓐᐦ ᐊᓂᑌ ᐃᔑ ᐯᒋ ᐅᑖᐦᒡ᙮ ᒫᔅᑰᒡ
ᐅᐦᒋᔥᑰ ᒌ ᐊᔭᒥᐦᐄᑰᑯᐸᓀ ᐊᐧᐁᔫᐦ ᐁᔅᒄ ᐁᒌ
ᐅᔅᒋᓃᒎᐧᐁᔨᐦᑖᑯᓯᑦ, ᓇᒧᐃ ᒋᐹ ᐅᐦᒋ ᐃᔥᐱᔥ
ᐋᐦᐧᑳᒋᐸᔨᓂᔫ ᑳ ᔩᐧᐋᑲᒥᐦᐧᑫᑦ ᑲᔦ ᐁᔅᒄ
ᓈᓂᑑ ᒋᐹ ᐊᔮᐤ ᐊᓂᔫ ᐅᔅᑳᑦ ᑳ ᒋᒥᔑᑲᓅᔨᒡ
ᑲᔦ ᐁᔅᒄ ᒋᐹ ᐊᔮᐤ ᑎᐱᔦᐤ ᐅᑌᐦᑕᑯᓰᐦ ᑲᔦ
ᐅᐦᐹᐱᑯᓰᒻ᙮ ᐋᔥᑰ ᐯᐦᑕᒻ ᒉᐧᑳᔫ ᓂᑕᒧᒄ

le territoire. Il enseigne à son fils les méthodes traditionnelles du territoire afin qu'il sache que même une jambe de robot et des organes transplantés ne peuvent l'empêcher de vivre sur le territoire si c'est ce qu'il désire. Il chasse et ramène de l'orignal et autres gibiers à la maison, puis il les cuisine. Il fait du sport quand il le peut. Le bas de son dos est souvent douloureux, à cause du travail supplémentaire qu'il doit fournir pour compenser sa jambe artificielle, et son pied en chair et en os est parfois enflé à cause de tout cet exercice. Cependant, l'exercice est nécessaire à ce qu'il demeure en bonne santé, donc Jack s'y attèle. Lorsqu'il est stressé par la vie en général, il parle avec un aîné, et lorsqu'il est stressé par le travail, il parle à un psychologue pour que le stress ne s'accumule pas en lui.

living on the land if it's what you want to do. He hunts and brings home moose and other game, and he cooks it up. He exercises when he can. His lower back often aches from the extra work it has to do with an artificial leg and his flesh-and-blood foot sometimes gets swollen from all the exercise, but exercise is what has to happen if he wants to stay healthy, and so Jack does it. When he's stressed out about life in general, he talks with an Elder, and when he's stressed out about work, he talks to a psychologist so the stress doesn't bottle up inside.

Parfois, il pense à de la marde. Il en a entendu un tas au fil des ans. Peut-être que si quelqu'un avait été direct avec lui quand il était plus jeune, son diabète ne serait-il pas devenu aussi grave et peut-être aurait-il encore sa jambe, son rein et son pancréas d'origine. Parfois, il tombe encore sur de la marde. Un conseiller lui a dit il n'y a pas longtemps qu'il devait

Sometimes he thinks about bullshit. He heard piles of it over the years. Maybe if someone had been direct with him when he was younger, his diabetes would not have become so severe and he might still have his original leg and kidney and pancreas. Sometimes he still runs into bullshit. A counsellor told him not long ago that he had to accept that his time

ᐋᔩᐱᒡ ᓂᒋᔥᑭᒻ ᒫᐧᑳᔮᐤ ᐋᑳ ᑖᐧᐹᒥᑭᓂᔮᒡ᙮ ᓂᒧᐃ ᓈᔥᒡ ᐧᐋᔥᑭᒡ ᐋᔪᐧᐃᒄ ᑳᐦ ᐄᑎᑯᑦ ᐹᔨᒄ ᐊᓂᔩᐦ ᒫ ᐧᐄᒋᐦᐄᑯᑯᐱᓈ ᐋᑳ ᓂᐦᑖ ᒦᓐ ᒫ ᒌᐦ ᐃᐦᑖᑦ ᐊᓂᑖᐦ ᓂᑑᐦᐆᔅᒌᐦᒡ, ᐋᑳ ᑭᔭᐧᐹ ᒌᐦ ᐃᐦᑎᒃ ᐊᐧᐋᓐ ᐊᓂᑖᐦ ᒫ ᒌᐦ ᐃᐦᑖᑦ ᐊᓂᑖᐦ ᓂᑑᐦᐆᔅᒌᐦᒡ ᒥᒄ ᐋᐦ ᐹᔭᑯᓂᔭᒡ ᐅᔅᑳᑦ᙮ ᓂᒥ ᒋᔅᑐᑖᐤ ᒫᒃ ᒥᒄ ᐱᔩᐱᐦᐧᑳᔭᑦ = ᐋᑎ ᐧᐃᔭᐧᐄᑦ ᐊᓂᑖᐦ ᐅᐦᒋ ᓂᑐᐦᑯᔭᓂᑭᒥᑯᐦᒡ ᒫ ᓂᑑᐦᐅᑦ᙮ ᐹᔭᑯᔭᒡ ᐊᓐ ᒫ ᒌᐦ ᐃᐦᑎᔭᓐ ᒫᐧᑳᓐ ᐋᐦ ᐹᐦᑎᒥᓐ ᒫᐧᑳᓐ ᐋᐅᒄ ᒌᔭ ᒫ ᒌᐦ ᐧᐄᒌᐦᐄᓯᔭᓐ᙮

ᓂᒧᐃ ᓈᔥᒡ ᐧᐋᔥᑭᒡ ᑳ ᑯᐧᑳᒋᒥᑯᑦ ᐊᐧᐋᔭᐤᐦ, ᐊᔥᑎᑖᔭᐦᑖᓐ ᐋ ᒦᓐ ᐋᐦ ᒥᔭᑭᐧᐃᔭᓐ ᐊᑎᑎᐤ ᒫ ᒌᐦ ᒥᔪᐱᒫᑎᓯᔭᓐ ᑭᔩᐦ ᒥᔪᐱᔭᔭᓐ ᒋᐱᒫᑎᓰᐧᐃᓂᐦᒡ᙮ ᓂᒧᐃ ᑏᐧᐋᐦᒡ ᐅᐦᒋ ᒌᐦ ᓂᔥᐧᑳᐅᔑᐦᐋᐤ᙮

"ᓂᒧᐃ ᑭᔭᐧᐹ ᓈᐦᐋᐤ ᐊᓐ ᓂᑎᑖᔭᐦᑖᔭᐦᑖᓐ," ᐄᑖᐤ, "ᑭᔭᐧᐹ ᑳ ᐧᐄᒋᐦᐄᑦ ᐱᒫᒋᐦᐃᐧᐋᓯᐤ , ᒥᒄ ᐧᐋᔅ ᐧᐹᔥᑎᐤ ᓂᑎᑖᔭᐦᑎᐧᒫᓐ᙮"

ᓂᒧᐃ ᒋᔑᐧᐋᔒᔥᑎᐧᐋᐤ ᐊᓂᔩᐦ ᓂᑐᐦᑯᔭᓐᐦ ᓈᔥᒡ ᒥᐦᒫᐧᑖᐤ ᐋᐦ ᒌᐦ ᐧᐃᓂᐱᔭᔭᒡ, ᑭᔩᐦ ᓂᒧᐃ ᐧᐄᐦ ᑎᐹᔅᑯᓈᐤ ᐊᐧᐋᔭᐤᐦ ᐅᐦᒋ ᐋᑳ ᑯᐃᔅᒄ ᐅᐦᒋ ᐄᔑ ᐧᐄᒋᐦᐄᑯᑦ᙮ ᐹᔭᐧᑳᐤ ᒌᐦ ᐄᑖᐤ ᐅᐧᐄᒫᐧᐋᑭᓐᐦ, ᒌᐦ ᑎᐹᔅᑯᓂᒫᑦ ᐊᓂᔩ ᑳ ᒥᓂᔑᑭᓂᐧᐃᐧᐃᔭᒡ ᐅᔅᑳᑦ, ᒌᐦ ᐱᔅᒋᔩᒫᑦ ᒫᒃ, ᒥᒄ ᐊᑎᑎᐤ ᓓᐧᐃᔩᓐᐦ ᒋᐱᐦᒌᐦ ᒥᔩᑭᓂᐆ, ᐊᓂᔩᐦ ᒫᒃ ᒌᐦ ᒥᔩᑭᓂᐧᐃᑦ ᐊᓂᔩᐦ ᒥᔥᑏᐦ ᓓᐧᐃᔩᓐᐦ ᐋᑯᑖᐦ ᒥᒄ ᒋᐱᐦᒌᐦ ᐄᑖᐱᒋᐦᐋᐤ ᐋᐦ ᒥᓂᐦᐧᑳᐧᐋᒫᑦ ᑭᔩᐦ ᐋᐦ ᐃᔩᔭᒥᓯᑦ, ᑭᔩᐦ ᐋᑯᑎᐦ ᒋᐱᐦᒌᐦ ᐅᐦᒋᐱᔭᔭᐤ ᐊᑎᑎᐤ ᒥᔥᑏᐦ ᓂᓈᐦᑭᐤ

ᐁ ᐄᓈᓅᔭᒡ᙮ ᓇᒧᐃ ᐧᐁᔅᑲᒡ ᒌ ᐃᑎᑰ ᐁ ᐊᔭᒥᐦᐄᑯᑦ ᐊᐧᐁᔫ ᑫᐧᐋ ᒋᔅᑫᔭᐦᑕᐦᒃ ᐁᑳ ᓵᔅ ᒋᓀᐅᔥ ᑫᒌ ᐃᐦᑖᑦ ᓅᐦᒋᒦᐦᒡ, ᓈᐯᐤ ᑮᐸ ᐁ ᓇᐸᑌᑳᑌᑦ ᓇᒧᐃ ᒋᐹ ᐅᐦᒋ ᓂᑑᐦᐆ᙮ ᒥᒄ ᒌ ᐹᐦᐱᐦᐧᑫᔫ ᐅᔫ ᑳ ᐄᑎᑯᑦ = ᑳ ᐊᑎ ᐧᐄᐧᐄᑦ ᐊᓂᑕ ᓂᑐᐦᑯᐃᓂᑲᒥᑯᐦᒡ ᑳ ᓂᑑ ᓂᑑᐦᐅᑦ᙮ ᐊᐧᐁᓐ ᐁᐧᐄ ᐧᐄᒋᐦᐄᓰᑦ ᑖᐹ ᒋᑲ ᐅᐦᒋ ᐋᐸᑕᐦᑕᐧᐁᐤ ᐊᐧᐁᔫ ᐁᑳ ᒧᔩᒻ ᐃᑎᑯᑦ ᑫᐧᑳᔫ᙮

ᐁᒄ ᒦᓐ ᓇᒧᐃ ᐧᐁᔅᑲᒡ, ᒌ ᑲᐧᑫᒋᒥᑰ ᐊᐧᐁᔫ ᐁ ᐃᑌᔭᐦᑕᒧᐧᑫ ᒧᐧᐁᐦᒡ ᑳᐤ ᐁᒌ ᒥᔩᑲᓅᑦ ᐁᑎᑑ ᑫᒌᔑ ᐱᒫᑎᓰᑦ ᐊᓂᔫ ᐁ ᐅᔅᒋᓯᔭᒡ ᐅᑌᐦᑕᑯᓰ ᑲᔦ ᐅᐦᐹᐱᑯᓰᒻ᙮ ᐧᐁᐃᐱᔅᒌᔥ ᒌ ᒫᒥᑐᓀᔭᐦᑕᒻ ᐅᔫ᙮

ᐁᒄ ᑳ ᐃᐧᑌᑦ, "ᓇᒧᐃ ᑮᐸ ᐯᑦ ᓈᔥ ᐁᑎᑑ ᒋᓀᐅᔥ ᑫᒌ ᐱᒫᑎᓯᔮᓐ ᓂᑎᑌᔭᐦᑌᓐ, ᐅᑌᐯᓕᐦᒋᑫᐤ ᓂᒌ ᓈᑕᒫᒄ ᒥᒄ ᒫᒃ ᑫᑳᑦ ᐧᐁᓵ ᓅᐦᑑ"᙮

ᓇᒧᐃ ᑮᐸ ᒋᓯᐧᐋᔒᔥᑕᐧᐁᐤ ᓂᑐᐦᑯᐃᓐᐦ ᐊᓂᔫ ᐁᒌ ᐧᐋᐧᐊᓂᐸᔭᔭᒡ ᑖᓐ ᑳ ᐃᔑ ᓇᓂᑕᐦᑯᐦᐄᑯᑦ ᑲᔦ ᓇᒧᐃ ᐧᐃᔩᔅᑯᓂᒉᐅᑲᒥᑯᐦᒡ ᐧᐄ ᐲᐦᑕᑲᐦᐁᐤ ᓂᑐᐦᑯᐃᓐ ᐁᑳ ᒧᔩᒻ ᐅᐦᒋ ᐃᐦᑑᑖᑯᑦ ᓓᓕᔩᔫ ᑫᒌ ᐅᐦᒋ ᒥᔅᑲᐦᒃ᙮ ᒌᐦ ᐄᑌᐤ ᐯᔨᒄ ᐅᐧᐄᑫᐧᐋᑲᓐᐦ, ᒌᐦ ᐧᐃᔩᔅᑯᓈᐅᒋᐸᓀ ᐊᓐ ᓂᑐᐦᑯᐃᓐᐦ ᐁᑳ ᒧᔩᒻ ᐅᐦᒋ ᐃᐦᑑᑕᐅᑦ ᐁᔅᒄ ᐁᒌ ᐋᔩᔩᓐ ᓂᔅᑳᑦ ᒥᔅᑕᐦᐄ ᓂᐹ ᒥᔅᑫᓐ ᓓᓕᔩᐤ, ᓈᓂᑑ ᐱᔑᒄ ᓂᐹ ᒌᔥᐧᑫᐧᐋᑫᓐ ᐊᓐ ᓓᓕᔩᐤ ᐁ ᒥᓂᐦᐧᑫᔩᓐ᙮ ᑲᔦ ᒫᒃ ᐁᑎᑑ ᓈᓂᑑ ᓇᒧᐃ ᓂᐹ ᐅᐦᒋ ᒋᐦᑳᐧᐋᒋᐸᔭᓐ ᓂᔩᐦᒡ, ᒌ

accepter que son temps dans le bois était révolu, qu'un unijambiste ne devrait pas d'adonner à la chasse. Jack a souri poliment, puis il a quitté la clinique pour aller chasser. La façon de gérer la marde, c'est de s'aider soi-même.

in the bush was over, that hunting was not something a one-legged man should do. Jack smiled politely – then left the clinic to go hunting. The way to deal with bullshit is to help yourself.

Il n'y a pas longtemps, quelqu'un lui a demandé s'il avait l'impression que ses nouveaux organes lui avaient donné une seconde chance. Il y a réfléchi pendant un moment.

Not long ago, someone asked him if he felt like his new organs had given him a second chance. He thought about it for a while.

« Pas une seconde chance, précisément, a-t-il dit. J'ai l'impression que le Seigneur m'a entendu. Mais un peu trop tard ».

"Not a second chance, exactly," he said. "I feel like the Lord came through. But a little too late."

Il n'est pas en colère contre les médecins qui ont fait tant d'erreurs, et il ne veut poursuivre personne pour faute professionnelle. Il a dit un jour à un ami que, s'il avait intenté un procès à l'époque où sa jambe a dû être amputée à cause d'une erreur d'un médecin, il aurait simplement eu plus d'argent, qu'il aurait dépensé pour boire et faire la fête, ce qui aurait entraîné encore plus de problèmes de santé. Il n'est pas non plus en colère

He's not angry at the doctors who made so many mistakes, and he doesn't want to sue anyone for malpractice. He told a friend once that, if he had sued back when his leg had to be amputated because of a doctor's mistake, he would just have had more money, which he would have spent on more drinking and partying, which would have led to even more health problems. Nor is he angry at his bosses who didn't want the liability of

ᒑ ᒌᐦ ᐋᐦᑯᓯᑦ ᐅᔮᐦᒡ ᑮᔮᐦ ᐅᒥᑐᓈᔨᐦᒋᑭᓂᐦᒡ᙮ ᓂᒧᐃ ᑮᔮᐦ ᒋᔑᐧᐋᔒᔥᑎᐧᐋᐤ ᐊᓂᔮᐦ ᑳ ᐅᒋᒫᒥᑦ ᐋᑳ ᐅᐦᒋ ᓂᐦᐋᔨᒥᑯᑦ ᒑ ᒌᐦ ᐋᐱᑎᓰᑦ ᐊᓂᑖᐦ ᐧᐃᔨᐧᐄᑎᒥᐦᒡ᙮ ᓂᒧᐃ ᑮᔮᐦ ᒋᔑᐧᐋᐦᐄᑰ ᐊᓂᔮ ᓈᔥᒡ ᐋᐦ ᒌᐦ ᐧᐋᐦᑎᒋᔥᑖᑯᓂᔨᒡ ᒥᔅᑳᑎᐦᑳᓂᔨᐤ ᑳ ᒥᔮᑭᓂᐧᐃᑦ ᐊᓂᑎᐦ ᑳᐦ ᐅᐦᒋᐱᔨᔨᒡ ᐊᑎᑎᐤ ᒑ ᒌᐦ ᒫᔮᑎᓂᔨᒡ ᐊᓂᔮ ᐅᔅᑳᑦ ᐋᑯᐦ ᒦᓐ ᑳ ᐄᔑᓈᑯᓂᔨᒡ ᒦᓐ ᐊᑎᑎᐤ ᒑ ᒫᒋᔑᑭᓂᐧᐃᐧᐃᔨᒡ ᐊᓂᔮ ᐅᔅᑳᑦ᙮ ᐊᓂᑖᐦ ᓃᔥᑖᒥᐦᒡ ᐧᐄᐦ ᐄᑖᐱᐤ, ᑯᐃᔅᒄ ᒑ ᒌᐦ ᐄᔑ ᐧᐄᒋᐦᐄᐧᐋᐱᔨᐦᑖᑦ ᐱᒫᑎᓰᐧᐃᓂᔨᐤ ᑮᔮᐦ ᑯᑎᒃᐦ ᐊᐧᐋᔨᐤᐦ ᒑ ᒌᐦ ᐧᐄᒋᐦᐋᑦ᙮

ᐋᑯᑖᐦ ᐋᑖᐱᑎᓰᑦ ᐋᐦ ᐊᔨᒥᐦᐋᑦ ᒑ ᒌᐦ ᐧᐄᒋᐦᐄᓯᔨᒡᐦ ᐊᐧᐋᔨᐤᐦ ᑮᔮᐦ ᒑ ᒌᐦ ᐊᔨᒥᐦᐋᑦ ᐊᓂᔮ ᐊᐧᐋᔨᐤᐦ ᐋᐦ ᒫᒥᑐᓈᔨᐦᑎᒥᔨᒡ ᑮᔮᐦ ᐋᐦ ᑯᐧᑳᑖᔨᐦᑎᒥᐦᐄᑯᔨᒡᐦ ᒑ ᒌᐦ ᐃᔮᔦᐧᐃᐦᑖᔨᒡᐦ ᐅᐱᒫᑎᓰᐧᐃᓂᔨᐤ ᐊᓂᑖᐦ ᐗᐧᓵᓂᐲᐦᒡ, ᑮᔮᐦ ᐧᐄᑎᐱᐦᒐᒨ ᐅᔮ ᐋᐦ ᐋᐱᔥᑎᑭᓂᐧᐃᐧᐃᔨᒡ ᐅᑖᐦ ᐄᔨᔨᐤᐦ ᑮᔮᐦ ᐄᔅᒌᒫᐤᐦ ᐋᐦ ᒫᒨᐱᔥᑎᑭᓂᐧᐃᐧᐃᔨᒡ ᐅᐦᒋ ᐅᔮ ᐅᑎᐦ ᑯᐯᒃ ᑮᔮᐦ ᒑᐱᓄᐧᑖᑫ ᑮᔮᐦ ᐧᐄᔨ ᑖᐦᒋᔥᑭᐧᐋᐤ ᐊᓂᔮᐦ ᓈᑳᓂᐱᔥᑎᒥᔨᒡᐦ ᐅᑖᐦ ᐄᑖᐦᒐ ᐊᑎᒫᐲᓯᒼ ᐊᓂᑎᐦ ᒑ ᒌᐦ ᐅᐦᒋ ᓂᑳᓂᑭᓂᐧᐃᐧᐃᔨᒡ ᐊᓂᔮ ᐋᐦ ᐄᑖᔨᐦᑎᐦᒡᐦ ᐊᐧᐋᓂᒌ ᐧᐄᔨᐧᐋᐤ ᒑ ᒌᐦ ᐃᔮᔦᐧᐃᐦᐄᓯᒡ᙮ ᐊᓂᑖᐦ ᑮᔮᐦ ᐄᔨᔨᐤ ᓂᑐᐦᑯᔨᓈᐱᑎᓰᐧᐃᓂᔨᐤ ᐋᐦ ᐅᐦᒋ ᐱᒥᐱᔨᐦᑖᑭᓂᐧᐃᐧᐃᔨᒡ ᐊᓂᑎᐦ ᓂᔮᓈᑭᒋᐦᐋᑭᓂᐅᐧᐃᒡ ᐊᐧᐋᓂᒌ ᐋᑳ ᒌᐦ ᑖᐱᐧᐄᒋᐦᐄᓯᒡ ᐅᐦᒋ ᐋᐦᑯᓯᐧᐃᓂᔨᐤ ᐋᐦ ᐄᐦᑐᑖᑯᒡ, ᐧᐄᔨ ᒑᒃ ᑮᔮᐦ ᐧᐄᐤᐦ ᐋᐦ ᐧᐄᒋᐦᐄᑯᑦ ᑭᓂᐧᐋᔨᒫᐧᐃᒡ ᐊᐧᐋᔑᔥᐦ ᐧᐋᔨᐱᔥᒌᔥ ᐋᑳ ᒌᐦ ᐧᐄᒋᒫᔨᒡᐦ ᐅᓃᒋᐦᐄᑯᔨᐤᐦ ᑮᔮᐦ ᐋᐅᒄ ᐹᔨᒄ

ᐃᑌᐤ᙮ ᓇᒧᐃ ᑲᔦ ᒋᔑᐧᐋᐦᐄᑰ ᐊᓂᔫᐦ ᑳ ᐅᒋᒫᒥᑦ ᐊᐧᐁᔫᐦ ᑳ ᐸᒋᔥᑎᓂᑯᑦ ᐊᓂᑌ ᐁ ᒋᒥᐦᐋᐦᑎᐧᑳᓄᔨᒃ ᑳᒌ ᐋᐸᑎᓯᑦ᙮ ᓇᒧᐃ ᑲᔦ ᒋᓯᐧᐋᐦᐄᑰ ᐊᓂᔫᐦ ᐊᐧᐁᔫᐦ ᐁᑳ ᑳ ᒥᐧᔮᔨᒃ ᐅᔅᑳᑎᐦᑲᓂᔫ ᑳ ᒦᑯᑦ ᓈᔅᒡ ᐁᒌ ᐋᐦᑯᐦᐄᑯᑦ ᒉᒃ ᑳ ᐊᑎ ᐃᔑᓈᑯᓂᔨᒡ ᐁᑎᑑ ᒦᓐ ᒉᒌ ᒋᒥᔑᑲᓄᔨᒡ ᐊᓂᔫ ᐅᔅᑳᑦ᙮ ᓇᒧᐃ ᐧᐄᐦ ᑲᓇᐧᐋᐸᐦᑕᒼ ᐅᑖᐦᒡ ᑖᓐ ᑳ ᐯᒋ ᐃᔅᐸᔨᑦ, ᒋᔑᓀ ᐁ ᒥᔦᔨᐦᑕᐦᒃ ᐅᐱᒫᑎᓰᐧᐃᓐ ᐁᐅᒄ ᐧᐋ ᒪᒣᒋᒥᓇᐦᒃ ᑲᔦ ᐧᑳᔥᑦ ᒉᒌᔑ ᐧᐋᐧᐄᒋᐦᐄᐧᐁᑦ ᐊᓂᑌ ᓀᑐᐧᐁᔨᐦᑖᑯᓯᑦ ᐁᑯᓐ ᐧᐋ ᐃᐦᑎᑦ᙮

ᐊᓄᐦᒌᔥ ᒫᒃ ᐁᐅᒄ ᐁ ᐄᑖᐸᑎᓯᑦ ᐧᐋᔅᐧᐋᓂᐲ ᐅᔅᒋᓃᒎ ᐁ ᒥᑯᔥᑳᑌᔨᐦᑕᒥᐦᐄᑯᔨᒃ ᒉᐧᑳᔦ ᐅᐱᒫᑎᓰᐧᐃᓂᔨᐦᒃ ᐁ ᐊᔨᒥᐦᐋᑦ ᑲᔦ ᐋᐸᑎᓰᐦᑲᐦᑕᒼ ᑖᓐ ᒉ ᐃᔑ ᐧᐋᐧᐄᒋᐦᐋᑲᓅᑦ ᐅᔅᒋᓃᒎ ᐁᑲ ᒉᒌ ᑕᐦᑯᐦᑖᑦ ᐅᐱᒫᑎᓰᐧᐃᓐ, ᑲᔦ ᐊᓯᑖᐴ ᐊᓂᑕ ᐁ ᒫᒨᐱᔥᑖᑲᓅᐦᒡ ᐆ ᐋᐸᑎᓯᐧᐃᓐ ᐁ ᐧᐄᑕᐸᒥᑯᑦ ᐄᓅᐦ ᑲᔦ ᐄᔅᒌᒣᐤᐦ ᐅᑕ ᑰᐯᒃ ᑲᔦ ᒑᐸᑫᐧᑖᑫ, ᑲᔦ ᐧᐄᒋᐦᐄᐧᐁᐤ ᐊᓂᔦ ᓇᓈᐦᑰ ᐁ ᐃᔑ ᐧᐄᒋᐦᐋᑲᓅᐧᑖᐤ ᐊᐧᐁᓂᒌ ᐁᑳ ᒉᒌ ᑕᐦᑯᐦᑖᐧᑖᐤ ᐅᐱᒫᑎᓰᐧᐃᓂᐧᐋᐤᐦ᙮ ᐊᑐᔅᑲᐧᐁᐤ ᒥᔦᐱᒫᑎᓰᐧᐃᓂᔦ ᑳ ᓇᓈᑲᒋᐦᑖᔨᒡ ᒥᓯᐧᐁ ᐅᑌ ᐃᔨᔨᐤ ᐊᔅᒌᐦᒡ ᐁ ᐧᐄᒋᐦᐋᑲᓄᔨᒡ ᐊᓂᔦ ᐊᐧᐁᔫᐦ ᐁ ᐃᐦᑕᑯᓂᔨᒡ ᒉᐧᑳᔦ ᐁᑳ ᒌ ᐃᐦᑑᑕᒫᓯᔨᒡ, ᑲᔦ ᒫᒃ ᑖᐱᔅᑯᓐ ᐧᐄᔭ ᐁᒄ ᒫᒃ ᐧᐄᒋᔅᐧᑫᐤ ᑲᓇᐧᐁᔨᒣᐅᒡ ᐊᐧᐋᔕ ᒣᐧᑳᒡ ᐁᑳ ᒌ ᐊᔮᐅᑲᐧᐃᔨᒡ ᐅᓃᒋᐦᐄᑯᔦ᙮ ᓀᔅᑕ ᑲᔦ ᐁᐅᒄ ᐁ ᐄᐦᑎᑦ ᐁ ᐊᔓᐧᐋᐸᐦᑕᐦᒃ ᒉᒌ ᐧᐄᔔᒫᑲᓅᑦ ᐁ ᓂᑐᐧᐁᔨᐦᑖᑯᓯᑦ ᒉᒌ ᓈᑕᒫᒉᑦ ᐅᔅᒋᓃᒎ ᐁᐧᐄ ᐧᐄᒋᐦᐋᑲᓄᔨᒡ᙮

contre ses patrons qui ne voulaient pas de la responsabilité de son travail dans le domaine forestier. Il n'est même pas en colère contre les personnes qui lui ont fourni une prothèse bon marché, qui n'a fait qu'irriter davantage sa jambe et a entrainé une seconde amputation. Ce qu'il veut, c'est aller de l'avant, continuer à vivre la belle vie qu'il a, apporter une contribution significative.

having him working in forestry. He's not even angry at the people who provided a cheap prosthesis that only irritated his leg further and led to a second amputation. What he wants is to move on, to continue to live the good life he has, to contribute in meaningful ways.

Il travaille comme conseiller et agent de prévention du suicide auprès des jeunes de Waswanipi, fait partie du conseil d'administration des L'Association Prévention Suicide Premières Nations et Inuits du Québec et du Labrador, et est co-président de la prévention du suicide dans la région. Il travaille également avec le Conseil cri de la santé pour protéger les moyens de subsistance des personnes handicapées. Enfin, sa femme et lui servent de famille d'accueil à des enfants et leur fournissent un foyer sûr lorsque ceux-ci ne peuvent pas être avec leurs parents, et il est de garde avec la Protection de la jeunesse.

He works as a counsellor and suicide prevention officer with the youth of Waswanipi, is on the Board of Directors for First Nations and Inuit of Québec and Labrador, and is the co-president of Suicide Prevention in the region. He also works with the Cree Board of Health to protect the livelihoods of people with disabilities, he and his wife foster kids and provide a safe home for them when they can't be with their parents, and he is on call with Youth Protection.

ᐊᐧᐋᓐ ᒥᒄ ᒑ ᒌᐦ ᐄᔑ ᒥᐧᑖᐦᑎᐧᐋᑭᓂᐧᐃᑦ ᐋᑳ ᒥᔪᐱᔭᒡᐦ ᐅᔅᒋᓃᒋᓲᐦ᙮

ᐊᓂᔮᐦ ᒫᒃ ᐱᔥᒡ ᐅᔅᒋᓃᒋᓲᐦ ᐃᔮᐱᑎᔒᔥᑎᐧᐋᑦ ᔖᔥ ᒥᔥᑏᐦ ᑭᔮᐦ ᒌᐦ ᐹᐦᑎᒥᔭᐤᐦ ᒑᐧᑳᔭᐤ ᐋᑳ ᑖᐧᐹᒥᑭᓂᔭᒡ᙮ ᐧᐄᔭ ᒫᒃ ᓈᔥᑖᐧᐹᐦ ᑯᐃᔅᒄ ᐄᔑ ᐧᐄᐦᑎᒧᐧᐋᐤ, ᑭᔮᐦ ᓂᒧᐃ ᑳᑐᐧᐋᐤ ᒑᐧᑳᔭᐤ, ᐋᔪᐧᐃᒄ ᐋᑖᑦ, “ᒫᐅᑖᐦ ᒑ ᒌᐦ ᐃᐦᑎᔭᓐ᙮ ᒥᔑᐤ ᒫᒃ ᐋᑳ ᐃᐦᑐᑎᒥᓈ ᐆ, ᒫᐅᑖᐦ ᒑ ᐄᔅᐱᔭᔭᓐ᙮” ᐧᐄᐦᑎᒧᐧᐋᐤ ᒑ ᒥᔪᓈᓈᑭᒋᐦᐄᓯᔭᒡᐦ, ᑯᐃᔅᒄ ᒑ ᐄᔑ ᒦᒋᓯᔭᒡᐦ, ᐋᑳ ᒑ ᒫᓯᐦᒑᔭᒡᐦ, ᑭᔮᐦ ᒫᒃ ᒥᒄ ᐊᓂᔭ ᒑᐧᑳᔭᐤ ᐊᓂᑎᐦ ᒑ ᒌᐦ ᐅᐦᒋ ᒥᔪᐱᔭᔭᒡᐦ ᐅᐱᒫᑎᓰᐧᐃᓂᐧᐋᔭᐦᒡᐦ ᒑ ᑯᒋᔥᑖᔭᒡᐦ᙮ ᐊᓂᔮᐦ ᒫᒃ ᐋᐦ ᐄᑖᑦ, ᐧᐃᔮᐱᐦᑎᔮᑦ ᐊᓂᔮ ᐅᔅᑲᑎᐦᑳᓐ ᑭᔮᐦ ᐋᑯᑎᐦ ᐧᐋᐦᒋ ᒌᐦ ᑖᐧᐹᐦᑖᑯᑦ᙮

ᐋᔥᒄ ᒨᔥ ᒋᔅᒋᓲᑎᑎᐧᐋᐤ ᐊᓂᔮᐦ ᐄᔭᔭᐤᐦ ᐊᓂᑖᐦ ᓂᑐᐦᑯᔭᓂᑭᒥᑯᐦᒡ ᐋᐦ ᐄᐦᑖᔭᒡᐦ ᐋᑳ ᐃᐦᑖᔭᐦᒡᐦ ᐊᐧᐋᔭᐤᐦ ᒑ ᒌᐦ ᐧᐋᐧᐄᒋᐦᐄᑯᔭᒡᐦ᙮ ᒑᒃ ᒫᒃ ᐊᓂᑖᐦ ᐄᔑ ᓃᔥᑖᒥᐦᒡ, ᒌᔖᐹᐧᐃᔭᒋᐦᐋ ᐊᓂᔮᐦ ᐅᑯᓯᔅ ᐦ ᑭᔮᐦ ᒌᐦ ᒋᔅᑯᑎᒫᓯᔭᒋᐦᐋ ᐊᓂᑖᐦ ᐱᑯᑎᔅᑭᒥᑳᐦᒡ ᐋᐦ ᐄᐦᑖᓂᐧᐃᐧᐃᔭᒡ, ᒑᒃ ᑭᔮᐦ ᐧᐄᐤᐦ ᐧᑳᐧᔖᓐ ᐊᓂᑖᐦ ᐧᒫᓐᑎᓅᐧᔮᑦ ᒋᑭ ᐄᔑ ᐋᐦᑎᐳᐧᐃᒡ ᐊᓂᑎᐦ ᒑ ᒌᐦ ᐋᐱᑎᓲᑦ ᑭᔮᐦ ᒑ ᒌᐦ ᐧᐋᐧᐄᒋᐦᐋᑦ ᐊᐧᐋᔭᐤᐦ ᐋᐦ ᐋᔭᒥᐦᐋᑦ ᑭᔮᐦ ᒫᒃ ᒑ ᒌᐦ ᐄᐧᑖᔥᑎᒫᒑᑦ ᐊᓂᑖᐦ ᓂᑐᐦᑯᔭᓂᑭᒥᑯᐦᒡ᙮ ᐅᔮ ᒫᒃ ᒫᐧᑲᒡ ᐊᓅᐦᒡ ᐊᓂᑎᐦ ᐋᐦ ᐃᐦᑖᑦ ᐋᑯᑎᐦ ᐄᔑᓈᑯᓂᔭᒋᒑ ᒑ ᒌᐦ ᐃᐦᑖᑦ᙮

ᐊᓂᔫ ᒫᒃ ᐅᔅᒋᓃᒨ ᐧᐃᔮᐧᐄᒋᐦᐋᑦ ᐃᐦᑕᑯᓂᔫ ᑖᓐ ᐁ ᐃᔑ ᒣᒣᐦᒡ ᐄᑖᑲᓇᔭᒡ᙮ ᐁᒄ ᑏᐧᐁᐦᒡ ᐁ ᐄᑖᑦ, “ᐧᒫᐤ ᐧᐁᔥ ᑫ ᐃᐦᑎᔭᓐ᙮ ᐁᑳ ᐃᐦᑑᑕᒪᓀ ᒫᐤ ᑫ ᐃᔅᐸᔭᓐ”᙮ ᓲᐦᒋᒣᐤ ᑫᒌ ᒥᔫᓈᓈᑲᒋᐦᐄᓯᔭᒡ, ᒫᒃ ᑫᒌ ᐴᓂᔭᒡ ᐁ ᒥᓂᐦᐧᑫᔭᒡ ᒫᒃ ᑫᒌ ᓇᓈᑲᒋᐦᑖᔭᒡ ᑫᒌ ᒥᔫᒦᒋᓯᔭᒡ, ᒫᒃ ᑫᒌ ᐴᓂᔭᒡ ᐁ ᒫᔅᑫᔭᒡ, ᒫᒃ ᑫᒌ ᐃᐦᑑᑕᒥᔭᒡ ᐊᓂᔫ ᑫᐧᑳᔫ ᑫ ᐧᐄᒋᐦᐄᑯᔭᒡ ᐁᑎᑑ ᑫᒌ ᒥᔫᐸᔭᔭᒡ ᐅᐱᒫᑎᓰᐧᐃᓂᔭᐦᒡ᙮ ᑯᐃᔅᒄ ᐃᔑ ᐊᔭᒥᐦᐁᐤ, ᑌᑭᔅ ᐃᔑ ᐧᐄᐦᑕᒧᐧᐁᐤ ᑫ ᐃᐦᑎᔭᒡ ᑲᔦ ᑖᓐ ᑫ ᐃᐦᑎᔭᒡ ᐁᐧᐄ ᐧᐄᒋᐦᐄᓯᔭᒡ, ᑲᔦ ᐁ ᐄᑖᑦ ᐁᑳ ᑯᑕᒃ ᐊᐧᐁᔫᐦ ᑫᒌ ᐃᐦᑑᑕᒥᔭᒡ ᒥᒄ ᐧᐄᔭ ᑫᒌ ᐧᐄᒋᐦᐄᓯᑦ ᐊᐧᐁᓐ ᓰᒃ ᑯᒋᐦᑖᑌ᙮ ᐅᔫ ᒫᒃ ᐁ ᐄᔑ ᐊᔭᒥᐦᐋᑦ, ᐁᒄ ᑫ ᑲᓇᐧᐋᐸᐦᑕᒥᔭᒡ ᐊᓂᔫ ᐅᔅᑳᑦ ᐁᒄ ᑫ ᑖᐧᐯᐦᑖᑯᑦ ᐊᓂᔫ ᑳ ᐃᔑ ᐊᔭᒥᐦᐋᑦ᙮

ᐁᔅᒄ ᒫᒃ ᔮᐸᒡ ᒫᒥᑐᓀᔭᒣᐤ ᐊᓂᔫᐦ ᐄᓅ ᐋᐦᑯᓲᐅᑲᒥᑯᐦᒡ ᑳ ᐃᐦᑖᔭᐧᑖᐤ ᑳ ᐋᐦᑯᓲᐧᑖᐤ᙮ ᒌᔑ ᓂᐦᑖᐅᒋᔭᑫᓐᐦ ᒫᒃ ᐅᑯᔅ ᑲᔦ ᐁᑎᑑ ᒋᔅᑫᔭᐦᑕᒥᔭᑫᓐ ᐁ ᐃᔑ ᐱᒫᒋᐦᐅᓈᓄᔭᒡ ᓅᐦᒋᒦᐦᒡ ᐁᒄ ᒨᓕᔮᐦᒡ ᑫᐧᐄᔑ ᐋᐦᑐᑫᐧᑖᐤ ᒫᐧᐃ ᒋᑲᒌ ᒥᔅᑰ ᐋᐸᑎᓰ ᐁ ᐊᔭᒥᐦᐋᑦ ᐋᐦᑯᓲᐅᐄᓅᐦ ᒫᒃ ᑳ ᐄᐧᑌᔥᑕᒧᐧᐋᑦ ᑫᒌ ᐄᑖᐸᑎᓯᑦ᙮ ᐊᓅᐦᒌᔥ ᒫᒃ ᐁᑯᑦ ᑫ ᐃᐦᑖᑦ ᑖᓂᑕ ᐁ ᐃᐦᑖᑦ ᒣᐧᑲᒡ᙮

Les jeunes avec lesquels il travaille ont entendu un tas de marde eux aussi. Dès le départ, il leur dit donc franchement, « Écoute, voici ce que tu dois faire. Si tu ne le fais pas, voici ce qui va arriver ». Il leur dit de prendre soin d'eux-mêmes ou d'arrêter de boire, ou de manger plus sainement, ou d'arrêter de se battre, ou de faire tout ce qui est en leur pouvoir pour améliorer leur situation. Il leur dit la vérité, toute la vérité, y compris comment ils peuvent s'aider eux-mêmes, y compris que c'est à eux de rendre leur propre vie meilleure. Quand il dit cela, ils regardent sa jambe de robot et le croient.

Il pense encore à tous les Cris qui souffrent seuls dans les hôpitaux. Un jour, lorsque son fils aura grandi et qu'il aura appris tout ce qu'il doit savoir sur la vie sur le territoire, Jack et sa femme déménageront peut-être à Montréal, où il pourrait travailler comme conseiller et traducteur dans les hôpitaux. Pour l'instant, il se trouve là où il devrait être.

The youth he works with have heard piles of bullshit too. So he tells them direct, straight off the bat, "Look, this is what you gotta do. If you don't do it, this is what will happen." He tells them to look after themselves, or to stop drinking, or to eat healthier, or to stop fighting, or to do whatever they can do to improve their situation. He tells them the truth, all of it, including how they can help themselves, including that it's up to them to make their own lives better. When he says that, they look at his robot leg and believe him.

He still thinks of all the Cree who suffer alone in the hospitals. Eventually, after his son is grown and has learned about life on the land, Jack and his wife might move to Montréal where he might work as a counsellor and translator in the hospitals. For now, this is where he should be.

Syllabic Chart ᐄᔨᔨᐅᔥᑖᐤ

Tableau de caractères syllabiques ᐄᓅᔥᑌᐤ

ᐁ e		ᐃ i	ᐄ ii	ᐅ u	ᐆ uu	ᐊ a	ᐋ aa		ᐤ u	ᐦ h
	ᐌ we	ᐎ wi	ᐐ wii	ᐒ wu	ᐔ wuu	ᐗ wa		ᐙ waa		
ᐯ pe	ᐺ pwe	ᐱ pi	ᐲ pii	ᐳ pu	ᐴ puu	ᐸ pa	ᐹ paa	ᑆ pwaa	ᑉ p	
ᑌ te	ᑗ twe	ᑎ ti	ᑏ tii	ᑐ tu	ᑑ tuu	ᑕ ta	ᑖ taa	ᑤ twaa	ᑦ t	
ᑫ ke	ᑴ kwe	ᑭ ki	ᑮ kii	ᑯ ku	ᑰ kuu	ᑲ ka	ᑳ kaa	ᒁ kwaa	ᒃ k	ᒄ kw
ᒉ che	ᒒ chwe	ᒋ chi	ᒌ chii	ᒍ chu	ᒎ chuu	ᒐ cha	ᒑ chaa	ᒟ chwaa	ᒡ ch	
ᒣ me	ᒬ mwe	ᒥ mi	ᒦ mii	ᒧ mu	ᒨ muu	ᒪ ma	ᒫ maa	ᒹ mwaa	ᒻ m	ᒧ mw
ᓀ ne	ᓉ nwe	ᓂ ni	ᓃ nii	ᓄ nu	ᓅ nuu	ᓇ na	ᓈ naa	ᓍ nwaa	ᓐ n	
ᓓ le	ᓜ lwe	ᓕ li	ᓖ lii	ᓗ lu	ᓘ luu	ᓚ la	ᓛ laa	ᓨ lwaa	ᓪ l	
ᓭ se	ᓶ swe	ᓯ si	ᓰ sii	ᓱ su	ᓲ suu	ᓴ sa	ᓵ saa	ᔂ swaa	ᔅ s	
ᔐ she	ᔗ shwe	ᔑ shi	ᔒ shii	ᔓ shu	ᔔ shuu	ᔕ sha	ᔖ shaa	ᔡ shwaa	ᔥ sh	
ᔦ ye	ᔯ ywe	ᔨ yi	ᔩ yii	ᔪ yu	ᔫ yuu	ᔭ ya	ᔮ yaa	ᔻ ywaa	ᔾ y	
ᕃ re	ᐧᕃ rwe	ᕆ ri	ᕇ rii	ᕈ ru	ᕉ ruu	ᕋ ra	ᕌ raa	ᐧᕌ rwaa	ᕐ r	
ᕓ ve	ᐧᕓ vwe	ᕕ vi	ᕖ vii	ᕗ vu	ᕘ vuu	ᕙ va	ᕚ vaa	ᐧᕚ vwaa	ᕝ v/f/ph	
ᕞ the	ᐧᕞ thwe	ᕟ thi	ᕡ thii	ᕢ thu	ᕣ thuu	ᕤ tha	ᕥ thaa	ᕦ thwaa	ᕪ th	